THE COMPLETE KETO DIET PLAN FOR BEGINNERS

The Complete Guide to Lose Weight and Reduce Inflammation with 2000 days of Recipes and 61-Day Meal Plan

By

Adam Bennet

Disclaimer

The information contained in this eBook is provided generally solely for general informational purposes. While we make every effort to keep the information up to date and correct, we make no express or implied representations or warranties for your outcome of any recipe found in this eBook. There are a number of factors that could contribute to you not achieving the desired result when preparing any recipe. You may not achieve desired results due to variations in elements such as ingredients, cooking temperatures, typos, errors, omissions, or individual cooking ability. You should always use your best judgment when cooking with raw ingredients and seek expert advice before beginning if you are unsure. Please review all ingredients prior to trying a recipe in order to be fully aware of the presence of substances which might cause an adverse reaction in some consumers.

Table of Contents

Introduction

Do you feel like you need to lose weight before you can start working on your body? Perhaps you've always thought about losing weight, but you've never actually committed to doing something about it. Overly regimented meal plans, outlandish exercise contraptions, and a miracle drug that promises to melt away fat without any physical exertion whatsoever; these are just some of the extreme methods for losing weight that have been proposed. When looking for help, you can choose from any number of these supposedly effective options from the dazzling, multibillion-dollar weight loss business.

If you've found this book, you probably have a good idea of what it takes to lose weight in a healthy way and keep it off for good. It's a known fact that eating less is the surest way to trim extra pounds.

Here's where the ketogenic diet excels and sets you free from the regular calorie restrictions of other diets to enjoy automatic, effortless fat burning.

You will almost certainly experience weight loss once you begin the ketogenic diet, but that is not the only benefit you will enjoy. There must be a long list of things you've always wanted to do but never got around to because you were too tired at the end of the day. On the ketogenic diet, you will have more energy for your regular activities; therefore it's time to get back to your old pastimes and interests. Clear thinking and incisive reasoning are additional benefits of the diet. Most people also notice an improvement in their health status as measured by improved lipid profiles, regulated blood sugar levels, and a reduced risk of cardiovascular disease.

The primary objective of this book is to provide you with the resources necessary to make the ketogenic diet more easily integrated into your lifestyle.

People often discover the hard way that the quality of their diet is directly proportional to the variety of foods it allows them to eat. Even the most ardent advocate of a specific diet plan would have trouble sticking to it if they were compelled to eat the same thing for breakfast, lunch, and supper every day. Here is where you should know that the ketogenic diet allows you a great deal of creative freedom in the kitchen, and it is the goal of this book to provide you with some of the most delicious and easy-to-prepare meals for your dining enjoyment.

The recipes included in this book are perfect for those just starting out on the ketogenic diet as well as those who have been following it for some time because they are delicious without taking up all of your time in the kitchen. The recipes are clear and concise, and they lay out the steps for making the meals in an easy-to-follow order.

Just by picking up this book, you've already demonstrated an interest in learning more about the ketogenic diet and its potential benefits. This keto diet cookbook will provide you with useful culinary inspiration to liven up your regular meals and providing best support on your ketogenic journey.

Chapter 1: The Secrets Of The Keto Diet

The ketogenic diet also called the keto diet, is not a new fad diet based on shaky science about nutrition. It has been around for a long time. The ancient Greeks used it as part of a whole-body treatment for epilepsy. In fact, it was a well-known way to treat epileptic seizures in children in the United States during the 1920s.

Unfortunately, this natural way of healing had to give way to the more immediate effects of modern pharmaceutical science.

The ketogenic diet is back in the spotlight, which is good news, and probably for very good reasons. You see, the whole point of the diet is to get your body to burn fat on its own so that it can get the energy it needs to get through the day. This means that both the fat you eat and the fat your body already has are now fuel stores that your body can use! It's no surprise that this diet really helps you lose weight, even in those stubborn places where fat is hard to get rid of. That could be one of the reasons you picked up this book and started looking into the ketogenic diet. Or, someone in your social circle may have told you that the keto diet actually normalizes blood sugar levels and improves cholesterol readings, and you are interested in that. How about stories about how people with type 2 diabetes were able to get rid of it just by following this diet? Or how the keto diet helped stop certain cancers or make the tumors shrink? We can't forget that the diet also lowers the risk of heart disease.

All of the above benefits of the ketogenic diet come mostly from a single important step in the diet. The goal is to get into ketosis.

1.1 Ketosis Know-How

In a state called "ketosis," the body makes molecules called "ketones." These are made by the liver. It gives energy to the organs and cells and can be used instead of glucose as a fuel source. In our traditional diet, which is high in carbs, most of our energy comes from glucose, which is made from the carbs we eat. Glucose is a quick source of energy, and insulin is needed to tell the cells to open up and let glucose flow in so that it can be used to fuel the mitochondria, which are the energy factories in our cells.

The more carbs we eat, the more glucose will be in our blood. This means that the pancreas needs to make more insulin so that the glucose in our blood can be used to make energy. When the body's metabolism is still working normally, the cells readily accept the insulin made by the pancreas.

This means that the blood sugar can be used as energy in an efficient way. The problem is that our cells can stop responding to insulin. This means that the pancreas has to pump more and more insulin into the body just to get the blood sugar levels back to normal.

Insulin resistance or Insulin de-sensitivity happens when the amount of glucose in the blood stays high for a long time. This is usually caused by eating carb-rich foods. Think of the cells in your body as a bouncer at a club where you have to pay a fee to get in. Here, you are glucose, and the price to get into the club is insulin. If you go to the club like everyone else, the bouncer won't notice anything out of the ordinary and won't raise the fee to get in. But if you show up almost every night yelling to get in, the bouncer will know how badly you need to get in and will raise the insulin fee to let the glucose in. The entry fee goes up and up over time, until the source of insulin, which in this particular scenario is the pancreas, can no longer make any. In this case, the person will be told they have type-2 diabetes, and the usual treatment is to take pills or insulin shots for the rest of their lives.

The most important thing here is that the body has glucose in it. When we eat a meal with a lot of carbs, which is easy to do in this day and era of fast food, our blood sugar goes up and insulin is released. Insulin turns the carbs into energy and stores any extra in fat cells. This is where the usual uproar starts, with glucose and insulin both being blamed for causing many diseases and the dreaded weight gain. Some books have made insulin and glucose out to be the source of all evil, which is not true. It would be much more accurate to say that the main cause of metabolic diseases and obesity that affect most of the developed world is the way we eat now.

The ketogenic diet is where the change for the better can be seen. The keto diet is a low-carb diet that focuses on eating a lot of fat. This plan is meant to help us eat less of the sugary and starchy foods that are so easy to find. Just for fun, sugar used to be used to keep things fresh. This is why many processed foods today have a lot of sugar in them, so they can last longer. Sugary foods have also been shown to cause the hedonic hunger response in the brain, which makes you eat for pleasure instead of because you're hungry. Studies have found that sugary treats affect parts of the brain that are also involved in drug and gambling addiction. Now you know why you can't stop putting those sugary candies in your mouth.

So we cut back on carbs, and fats step in to give the body the energy it needs to stay alive. On a standard ketogenic diet, you should get 75% of your daily calories from fats, 20% from proteins, and the remaining 5% from carbohydrates. We do this because, as you may recall, we want fats to be our main fuel source. Ketosis can only start when we cut back on carbs and eat more fat. Either we do it through a diet that can be used for a long time and is safe, or we starve ourselves into ketosis. Yes, you read that right. Ketosis is a natural process in the body that stores fat for times when food is scarce.

1.2 Is Keto A Starvation Diet?

This has been also talked around a lot in recent times, with some seeking to cast a negative light on the keto diet by means of linking it with starvation. To clarify, ketosis begins when the body realizes it does not have enough glucose and begins to break down fat for energy. The liver then uses fat storage to produce ketones, which are used to keep the body's cells and organs running on a steady flow of energy. It does not mean that on the keto diet, you are literally starving yourself! How can you be hunger when the meal plan provides you with 1,800 to 2,000 calories every day?

Ketosis was very useful for our ancestors who lived a hunter-gatherer lifestyle. During this time, agriculture wasn't widespread, so people had to rely on what they could find or hunt for sustenance. This meant that there might be times when we wouldn't eat for several days, so our systems would release insulin in response to ingested glucose in order to transport it to the organs that needed it and store any excess in fat cells.

When there was nothing to eat, the body went into ketosis and used its fat reserves for fuel. In this condition, our bodies produce hunger hormones like ghrelin lowered, and the hormones which control fullness, such leptin, find their levels boosted. When it senses that food is short, our bodies do all this to make sure we're as comfortable as possible despite the situation.

Now, in the present period, food is usually no more than a couple blocks away, if not a short drive in a car, so it's safe to assume that we won't encounter food shortages like our Paleolithic forebears did. But the processes and mechanisms that allowed them to live in our bodies are still active. That's why, on the keto diet, we try to limit our carbohydrate consumption while upping our fat intake. When we do that, the phase of ketosis is triggered, and we get to enjoy all the metabolic benefits which the diet imparts. You will not be hungry on a ketogenic diet because the fat we eat is also used to restore our body's fat stores.

It is at this time that some people begin to zero in on the billion dollar query. Why does almost everyone lose weight while on the keto diet if ingesting fats causes fat storage?

1.3 How Keto Helps In Weight Loss

When we start the ketogenic diet, one of the first things we always lose is most likely water weight. The body stores glucose as adipose fat, but it also stores a small amount of glucose as glycogen, which is mostly water. Glycogen is meant to give us the kind of quick bursts of energy we need when we run or lift weights. When we cut back on carbs, our bodies use glycogen as the first source of energy. This is why we lose water weight in the beginning. This first wave of weight loss can be a morale booster for many people, and it's a good sign of what's to come for people who stick with the keto diet. On a side note, it's easy to lose and gain water weight. This means that if someone starts to lose weight on the keto diet but then quits for some reason, their weight is likely to go back up once carbs become the main source of calories in their daily diet.

For those who stick with the ketogenic diet, what happens next is that the body's fat-burning system takes over. This is why many people lose weight so quickly on the ketogenic diet. The basic idea is still the same, which is that adipose fats are now used as energy sources by the organs and cells of the body. This makes fat loss and weight loss happen naturally.

The keto diet helps people lose weight in more ways than just by making them burn fat. People can lose weight better while on a diet because it makes them feel fuller after meals and make them feel less hungry. One of the oldest rules for losing weight has always been to eat less and move more. The whole point is to burn more calories than you take in, so that your body has to use its stored energy to make up for the difference. On paper, that sounds simple and easy, but anyone who has ever had to consciously stop eating when they were hungry knows that it can be as hard as climbing Mount Everest.

Because the hormones that control hunger and fullness are changed by the ketogenic diet, you can be sure that your hunger will go away on its own. Also, the food we eat while on a diet helps us lose weight. Sugary carbs are known to make you feel less full than fats and proteins. When we switch to a high-fat diet and cut back on carbs, we pretty much accomplish two things at the same time. Getting less carbs, especially sugary carbs, makes you less likely to eat just because you want to, not because you are hungry. Increasing the amount of fat you eat also makes you feel full much more quickly. This is one reason why many people on the keto diet say they can get by on two and a half meals or even just two meals a day without feeling hungry.

On the keto meal plan, we plan for a daily calorie intake of between 1,800 and 2,000 calories, so we don't really count calories to lose weight. When you're full and happy from your meals, those tiny, innocent-looking snacks won't be a big part of your life. Think about it: snacks like donuts, chips, and cakes are cut out because they make you more likely to give in to hedonistic hunger, which is mostly caused by sugary treats. That cuts a lot of extra calories that would have been turned into adipose fat tissue if you didn't do it.

To sum up, the ketogenic diet lets you eat what you want and doesn't limit calories like most other diets do. It also helps create effects that make you feel less hungry, so you don't have to deal with those awful hunger pangs! There are also no cravings for carbs, which can make it hard to stick to a diet. This lets us lose weight in a healthy way with as little trouble as possible in our daily lives. No calorie counters are needed, and you don't have to eat six to eight meals a day. Also, you don't have to do any weird or funny exercises. When you add that to the fact that keto high-fat meals make you feel full, hunger might start to feel like a stranger.

Being able to remember what real hunger feels like is also a good thing. When we eat a lot of carbs, our blood sugar levels tend to go up and down a lot, making us feel hungry. This happens because our cells become less sensitive to insulin over time. Sugar also makes people more likely to eat on the spot, which can really mess up a diet. When we cut back on carbs and eat more fats, we would have to pay close attention to any hunger pangs because they would be signs that our bodies need to refuel.

1.4 Important Tips For Ketogenic Diet

If you want to lose weight, eat a good keto breakfast

You should give yourself time to start the day off right. If you eat a good breakfast with protein and healthy fats in the morning, like egg muffins or an omelet, you will eat less during the day. Eating a healthy breakfast with few carbs can help restore your body's glucose levels in a big way, just like your car needs gas to run. You should eat foods that are high in protein, like nuts, milk, eggs and seeds. Skipping breakfast can change how you feel and how well you can think. It can also cause high blood pressure, high cholesterol, and hypertension. Studies have shown that people who don't eat breakfast are very tired during the day.

If you think you don't have time for breakfast, this collection of recipes might help you out. This book has easy breakfast ideas like egg muffins, omelette roll-up, low-carb pancakes, and more. You can also eat leftovers from dinner for breakfast. A casserole with bacon, eggs, and sharp cheese on top is a great way to relax for dinner or grab a quick breakfast on the go. If you don't have much time, it's a good idea to make breakfast ahead of time. For example, you can make chicken salad, lettuce wraps, or cheese crisps and store them in airtight containers for up to 3 days. You can make a vegetable and cheese gratin on Sunday morning. It's easy to reheat or you can eat it cold right out of the fridge. With the keto recipes, it's easy to make meal prep a regular part of your life. Don't forget that your body needs fuel right away in the morning.

So, eat breakfast in the first hour after you wake up. Breakfast is one of the most important parts of a healthy keto diet and a key to better health in general.

Learn to use the nutrition facts label

First of all, keep the carbs low. It will help you choose healthier foods that are good for your diet. Then, look for hidden sugars, which are a keto diet's "number one enemy." Most processed foods hide sugar because it makes foods taste better and helps them last longer. Raw sugar, sucrose, sugar syrup, brown sugar, invert sugar, high-fructose corn syrup, corn syrup, cane sugar, corn sweetener, Turbinado, fructose, dextrose, fruit juice concentrates, glucose, maltose, malt syrup, lactose, and Sorghum syrup are all common sweeteners. They don't add anything good to your meals in terms of health.

You should also stay away from caramel, cane juice, dextran, dextrin, beet sugar, barley malt, carob syrup, buttered syrup, diatase, date sugar, golden syrup, diatastic malt, Refiner's syrup, and ethyl maltol.

Statistics show that the average American eats at least 22 tsp. of added sugars or 64 pounds of sugar per year. When it comes to healthy keto sweeteners, you should choose one that is made from natural ingredients and does not contain chemicals. You should also choose a sweetener that is good for you and doesn't put you over your daily carb limit. Monk fruit and Stevia are natural sugar substitutes that are good for your health. Stevia is 300 times sweeter than sugar, but it has no effect on how much sugar is in the blood. Look for an organic and pure product when you buy stevia. Monk fruit has no calories and has been shown in studies to have powerful antioxidant and anti-inflammatory properties. It can help reduce inflammation and keep insulin tolerance in check.

Calculate net carbs

For a keto diet to work, you need to know how to figure out net carbs. In fact, net carbs are the carbs that our bodies can break down and use as fuel. Stay with the plan: Total carbs minus dietary fiber plus sugar alcohols equals net carbs. Dietary fiber and most sugar alcohols are carbs that can't be broken down by the body. Your liver doesn't turn carbs that can't be broken down into glucose. So, only starches and sugars are counted in net carbs.

That is, you don't have to count sugar alcohols like xylitol, mannitol, lactitol, and erythritol toward your carb limit. On the other hand, about 0.5 grams of carbs are in each gram of isomalt, sorbitol, glycerin or maltitol. Also, fiber is counted as a carb, but our bodies can't use it for energy because they can't process it. Most food labels will list them under "Dietary Fiber." By keeping insulin levels steady, soluble dietary fiber is a key part of controlling hunger. Also, learning about macronutrients and how they affect your body is the key to a healthy low-carb diet. So, you might want to figure out your net carbs instead of your total carbs. If you are just starting out, be aware of hidden carbs.

Learn how to build muscle while following keto diet

Building lean mass is important for a ketogenic diet to work because it will help you burn fat more efficiently. You can boost the size of your muscles by doing overhead presses, deadlifts, bench press and squats. For the best athletic performance, it's important to refuel your body with keto foods that are high in nutrients. Also, pay close attention to how many electrolytes you take in. Mushrooms, broccoli, spinach, and salmon are all examples of foods that are low in carbs and high in potassium. Avocados, almonds, and dark chocolate are all high in magnesium and low in carbs.

Consider energy density

In fact, the number of calories in a gram of food is called its "energy density." For a keto diet, it's best to eat mostly foods with a medium amount of calories and eat small amounts of foods with more calories. On the other hand, foods with a lower energy density have fewer calories per gram. They include stews, clear soups, and vegetables and simple green salads that are naturally high in water.

Eating real food

This means that on a ketogenic diet, you'll need to eat unprocessed, whole foods that are high in nutrients. It is very important to stay away from chemicals and junk food. Your life will be easier and your body will be healthier if you focus on organic, whole, grass-fed foods.

1.5 Benefits Of A Ketogenic Diet

Helps in losing weight

Weight loss and maintenance are possible with the ketogenic diet. If you stick to the diet, you won't have to worry about sudden weight gains or drops. This can't happen because of how ketosis works, and we're talking about normal meals, not seven or eight thousand calorie diets, which would definitely mess up the process of losing weight. If you eat too much, you can still gain weight.

Better concentration and mental clarity

The ketogenic diet lowers overall toxin levels because the brain shifts to using ketones as its primary fuel source. As a result, you'll see a marked enhancement in memory, reasoning, attention span, and other mental abilities.

People who eat a lot of processed carbs don't get the brain fog that people who eat less processed carbs do. This clearer thinking is also helped by the fact that ketones burn more efficiently as fuel.

Improve your energy levels and get rid of chronic fatigue

Instead of having energy levels that go up and down like a roller coaster, you'll have more energy that stays more or less the same as long as you eat when you're hungry. Due to the increased energy, chronic fatigue is also no longer a problem. Even if the tiredness is a sign of another illness, many people find that the keto diet makes it better, even if it doesn't go away completely.

Less oxidative stress

The ketogenic diet increases the amount of antioxidants in the body and reduces the amount of oxidation that the mitochondria of the body have to deal with. With more antioxidants in our bodies while on the keto diet, it's harder for free radicals to cause oxidative damage to our bodies. When there is less oxidation, our cells and organs tend to work better and last longer. This also means that there might be a chance to live longer, since oxidation, which is one of the main causes of aging, is slowed down a little bit by the ketogenic diet.

Brings down your inflammation

When you make sure you have the right amount of omega-3 fats, they help to lower the body's inflammatory response. This is good news for people with diseases that cause inflammation all the time. Also, if you cut back on carbs, you're likely to eat a lot less sugar, which will definitely help reduce inflammation as well.

Increase your energy and stop feeling tired all the time

Instead of your energy going up and down like a roller coaster, the ketone fuel in your body will give you more energy that stays more or less the same as long as you eat when you're hungry. Due to the increased energy, chronic fatigue is also no longer a problem. Even if the tiredness is a sign of another illness, many people find that the keto diet makes it better, even if it doesn't go away completely.

Moods will be better and more stable

When the body goes into ketosis, it makes ketones for energy. These ketones also help keep the balance between two brain chemicals called neurotransmitters: GABA also called gamma-aminobutyric acid, and glutamate. GABA is used to calm down the brain, while glutamate is used to wake up the brain. Keeping these two substances in the right balance is the key to a healthy and happy brain, and ketones help with that.

Natural suppression of hunger

This is another great thing about the keto diet that can help you lose weight. Now you can do that without getting crazy hunger pains.

Health benefits

Carbohydrates, which are found in harmful sugary meals and refined grains like bread, pasta, and white rice, are limited on a ketogenic diet. On the other hand, it advocates for eating foods high in quality protein (muscle-building fuel), beneficial fats, and nutritious vegetables. Numerous scientific researches have demonstrated the health benefits of low-carbohydrate diets. LDL cholesterol, blood sugar, HDL cholesterol, triglyceride, and weight loss were the primary outcomes measured.

Consuming fatty fish regularly (such as salmon and tuna) has been shown to reduce triglyceride levels and, in turn, the risk of stroke. The unsaturated fats found in foods like seeds, nuts, and unprocessed vegetable oils can also aid in reducing triglyceride levels. As an added bonus, limiting carb intake helps control insulin and blood sugar levels. In addition to helping with weight loss and performance in the gym, ketogenic diets can be used to treat a variety of serious medical issues.

A number of neurological conditions, including epilepsy in children, have responded well to the ketogenic diet. Metabolic syndrome is well treated with ketogenic diets.

Chapter 2: Complete Keto Diet Food List

The ketogenic diet is high in fat, has a moderate amount of protein, and has very few carbs. The body gets most of its energy from carbs, but on a strict ketogenic diet, less than 5% of the energy comes from carbs. When you eat less carbs, your body goes into a metabolic state called ketosis. Ketosis is when the body stops getting the supply of blood sugar provided from the food we eat and starts making body fat molecules also known as ketones from the stored body fat. These ketones are used as energy. Once the body is in state of ketosis, most cells will use ketone bodies for fulfilling the body energy until you begin eating carbohydrates again.

In the past, the ketogenic diet was only used in hospitals to help children with epilepsy stop having seizures. Emily Stone, M.S., RD, says that there is a lot of interest in how well the diet can help with other neurological conditions, diabetes, cancer, polycystic ovary syndrome (PCOS), high cholesterol, obesity, and heart disease. People also eat keto to lose weight.

Even if you know you need to eat a very low-carb, moderate-protein and high-fat diet, it can be hard to figure out what foods to eat. Here is a list of what you can eat on a ketogenic diet, what you should avoid, and what you can sometimes have.

2.1 Foods to Eat On a Ketogenic Diet

Here is a list of all keto-friendly, low-carb foods you can eat when you're on the keto diet.

Seafood and fish

Fish has a lot of B vitamins, selenium and potassium. It's also carb-free and protein-rich. Fatty fish like sardines, salmon, albacore tuna, mackerel, and others have a lot of omega-3 fats, which have been shown to lower blood sugar and make insulin work better. People who eat fish often are less likely to get chronic diseases and have better mental health. Try to eat at least two 3-ounce portions of fatty fish each week.

Low-carb veggies

Non-starchy vegetables are low in carbs and calories but high in many nutrients, like vitamin C and several minerals. They also have antioxidants that protect against free radicals that damage cells. Aim for vegetables that don't have a lot of starch and have less than 8 grams of net carbs per cup. Total carbs minus fiber equals net carbs. The list includes cauliflower, broccoli, green beans, zucchini, bell peppers, and spinach.

Cheese

Cheese is a great food for the ketogenic diet because its carb free and has a lot of fat. It has a lot of protein and calcium as well. But a 1-ounce slice of cheese has about 30% of the Daily Value for saturated fat, so if you're concerned about heart disease, consider portion size while consuming it.

Cottage cheese and plain Greek yogurt

Cottage cheese and yogurt are both high in protein and calcium. Plain Greek yogurt has only 5 grams of carbs and 12 grams of protein in a 5-ounce serving. Cottage cheese has 5 grams of carbohydrates and 18 grams of protein in the same amount. Studies have shown that protein and calcium can both make you feel full and less hungry. Cottage cheese and Higher-fat yogurts help you feel full longer, and the ketogenic diet includes full-fat foods.

Avocados

Choose fats that are good for your heart, like avocados, which have a lot of potassium and monounsaturated fat, a mineral that many Americans don't get enough of. There are 9 grams of carbs in half of a medium avocado, 7 of which are fiber. Switching from fats from animals to fats from plants, like avocados, can help lower cholesterol and triglycerides.

Poultry and meat

Meat is an important part of the ketogenic diet because as it provides lean protein. Poultry and meat have no carbs and are full of B vitamins and many important minerals like potassium, selenium, and zinc. Even though processed meats like bacon and sausage are allowed on the keto diet, eating too much of them isn't good for your heart and may make you more likely to get some types of cancer. Choose more fish, chicken, and beef and less processed meat.

Eggs

Eggs have a lot of antioxidants, minerals, B vitamins, and protein. Eggs have been shown to make hormones that make you feel fuller and keep your blood sugar levels steady. They also contain antioxidants like zeaxanthin and lutein, which protect your eyes and help, keep them healthy.

Nuts, seeds and healthy oils

Nuts and seeds are full of healthy monounsaturated and polyunsaturated fats, fiber, and protein. Also, they have very few net carbs. On the keto diet, coconut oil and olive oil are the two best oils to use. There is a link between the amount of oleic acid in olive oil and a lower risk of heart disease. Coconut oil has a lot of saturated fat, but it also has medium-chain triglycerides (MCTs), which can help make more ketones. MCTs may speed up your metabolism and help you lose weight and belly fat. When you eat healthy fats, you should watch how much you eat.

Berries

Berries have a lot of antioxidants, which help reduce inflammation and keep you from getting sick. They have few carbohydrates and a lot of fiber.

Unsweetened tea and coffee

Plain tea and coffee have no carbs, fat, or protein in them, so they are fine to drink on the keto diet. Researchers have found that drinking coffee lowers the chance of getting heart disease and type-2 diabetes. Tea has more antioxidants than coffee and less caffeine. Drinking tea may lower your risk of stroke and heart attack, help you lose weight, and boost your immune system.

Cocoa powder and dark chocolate

Check the label to see how many carbs they have because it varies depending on the type and how much you eat. Cocoa has been called a "superfruit" because it is full of antioxidants, and dark chocolate has flavanols, which may lower the risk of heart disease by keeping arteries healthy and lowering blood pressure.

2.2 Foods To Avoid On A Ketogenic Diet

Here is a list of foods you should avoid when you're on the keto diet.

Grains

Cereal, rice, crackers, bread, pasta, and beer are high carbs food. Even bean-made pasta and whole-wheat pasta are also full of carbs. You could try healthier low-carb alternatives like shirataki noodles or spiralized vegetables. Both sugary and healthy whole-grain breakfast cereals are high in carbohydrates and should be avoided or eaten only in small amounts. "On average, a slice of bread has 11 grams of carbs, so you could have one slice a day," says Dority. "But that would be a waste of all your carbs, and for the same amount of carbs, you could eat a LOT of vegetables."

Beer can be enjoyed on a low-carb diet, but only in small amounts. Dry wine and spirits are better choices, but you shouldn't drink much of anything.

High-sugar fruits and starchy vegetables

Starchy vegetables have more digestible carbs than fiber, so the ketogenic diet says to eat less of them. Corn, sweet potatoes, potatoes, and beets are all examples. Limit high-sugar fruits, which have more carbs and raise your blood sugar more quickly than berries.

Sweetened yogurts

Stay with plain yogurt to cut down on added sugars. When compared to regular yogurt, Greek yogurt has more protein and less sugar.

Juices

Fruit juice, whether it's natural or not, is full of carbs that break down quickly and raise your blood sugar. Just drink water.

Any kind of honey, syrup, or sugar

Sugar, honey, maple syrup, and other sugary foods should be avoided because they are high in carbs and low in nutrients.

Crisps and chips

Chips, crackers, and other processed grain-based snack foods are high in carbs and low in fiber, so you should stay away from them.

Chapter 3: Breakfast Recipes

3.1 Ham, Mushroom And Spinach Frittata

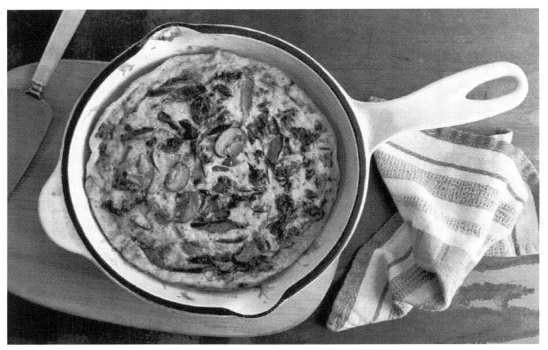

Preparation time: 4 mins

Cooking time: 9 mins

Servings: 2

Ingredients:

- 1 tsp. oil

- 1/3 cup ham, diced

- ½ cup chestnut mushrooms, sliced

- 4 medium eggs, beaten

- ½ cup spinach

- 1 tbsp. grated cheddar

Instructions:

- The grill should be heated to its highest setting. Over medium-high heat, heat the oil in a pan that can go in the oven. Add the mushrooms in and cook them for 2 minutes or until they are mostly soft. Stir in the spinach and ham, and cook for another minute, until the spinach has wilted. Add some salt and black pepper to taste.

- Turn down the heat and pour the sauce over the eggs. Cook without touching it for 3 minutes, or until most of the eggs are set. Sprinkle over the cheese and cook for 2 minutes under a grill. Serve and enjoy.

Nutritional values per serving: Calories: 226/kcal; Fat: 15 g; Carbs: 0 g; Fiber: 1 g; Protein: 22 g.

3.2 Zucchini Bread

Preparation time: 10 minutes

Cooking time: 50 minutes

Servings: 12

Ingredients:

- 3 oz. almond flour

- 1/2 tsp. salt

- 2 oz. coconut flour

- 2 tsp. baking powder

- 1/2 tsp. pepper

- 5 large eggs

- 1 tsp. xanthan gum

- 4 oz. cheddar cheese, grated

- 2/3 cup butter, melted

- 6 oz. bacon diced

- 6 oz. zucchini, grated

Instructions:

- Preheat the oven to 350°F.

- Mix the coconut flour, almond flour, baking powder, salt, pepper, and xanthan gum together in a large bowl. Blend well.

- Mix well after adding the eggs and melted butter.

- Mix in the zucchini, bacon, and 3/4 of the cheddar cheese.

- Put the mixture into a 9-inch ceramic loaf dish that has been greased. If you are using a meat dish, line it with parchment paper. Bake for 35 minutes, then take it out of the oven and sprinkle the rest of the cheese on top.

- Bake for another 10–15 minutes, or until the cheese has turned golden brown and a skewer comes out clean.

- Leave the bread for 20 minutes to cool down.

- Slice into 12 pieces and eat while still warm.

Nutritional values per serving: Calories 281 /kcal; Fat: 25 g; Carbs: 5 g; Fiber: 3 g; Protein: 9 g.

3.3 Tomato Baked Eggs

Preparation time: 10 mins

Cooking time: 50 mins

Servings: 4

Ingredients:

- 2 lb. ripe vine tomatoes

- 3 garlic cloves

- 3 tbsp. olive oil

- 2 tbsp. chopped parsley

- 4 large eggs

Instructions:

- Preheat the oven to 350°F. Depending on how large the tomatoes are, cut them into thick wedges or quarters, and then spread them out in a 1.5-liter oven-safe dish that isn't too deep. Peel the garlic, cut it into thin slices, and sprinkle it on top of the tomatoes. Sprinkle with olive oil, season with salt and pepper, and stir until the tomatoes are bright.

- Place the dish in the oven and bake for 40 minutes, or until the tomatoes have softened and started to turn brown.

- Make four holes in the tomatoes, crack an egg into each hole, and cover the dish with a piece of foil. Put it back in the oven for 5–10 minutes, or until the eggs are cooked the way you like. Sprinkle the herbs on top and serve with a green salad and thick slices of keto bread.

Nutritional values per serving: Calories: 204 /kcal; Fat: 16 g; Carbs: 7 g; Fiber: 3 g; Protein: 9 g.

3.4 Keto Bread

Preparation time: 10 mins

Cooking time: 50 mins

Servings: 12

Ingredients:

- ½ cup coconut oil, melted

- ¾ cup almond flour

- 1 tbsp. psyllium husk

- 1 tsp. baking soda

- 2 tsp. baking powder

- ½ cup milled seeds

- 1 tbsp. milled flaxseed

- 1½ tbsp. coconut flour

- Pinch of salt

- 1 medium courgette, grated

- 3 eggs, beaten

- 1 tbsp. apple cider vinegar

Instructions:

- Preheat the oven to 400°F. Grease and line a loaf tin and keep it aside.

- Mix all the dry ingredients together in a large bowl, and then set it aside.

- Put the eggs, coconut oil, courgette, and 1/2 cup of hot water in a separate large mixing bowl. Pour this mixture into the dry ingredients mixture and mix well. Add the apple cider vinegar and stir it in gently. Try not to mix the dough too much.

- Put the mixture into the loaf pan. Wet your fingers or the back of a spoon to smooth the top of the bread. After 20 minutes, turn the oven down to 350F and bake for another 30 minutes. Take the bread out of the oven and let cool for 10 minutes in the pan, then move to a cooling rack. Cut the bread into pieces and toast them in a pan or oven.

Nutritional values per serving: Calories: 220 /kcal; Fat: 19 g; Carbs: 3 g; Fiber: 3 g; Protein: 8 g.

3.5 Mushroom Brunch

Preparation time: 5 mins

Cooking time: 15 mins

Servings: 4

Ingredients:

- ½ lb. mushrooms

- 1 tbsp. olive oil

- 1 garlic clove

- 4 eggs

- 2 cups kale

- ½ tsp. salt

Instructions:

- Crush the garlic clove and slice the mushrooms. Heat the olive oil in a large pan that doesn't stick, and then cook the crushed garlic for 1 minute over low heat.

- Cook the mushrooms until they are soft. Now add the kale into the pan. If you can't fit all of the kale in the pan, add half, stir it until it wilts, and then add the rest. Once all of the kale has wilted, add salt.

- Now break the eggs in and cook them slowly for 2 to 3 minutes. Then, put the lid back on and cook for another 2 to 3 minutes, or until the eggs are done the way you like. Serve with keto bread and enjoy.

Nutritional values per serving: Calories: 154 /kcal; Fat: 11 g; Carbs: 1 g; Fiber: 2 g; Protein: 13 g.

3.6 Omelette Roll-Up

Preparation time: 5 mins

Cooking time: 10 mins

Servings: 1

Ingredients:

- 1 large egg

- 2 tbsp. tomato salsa

- 1 tsp. olive oil

- 1 tbsp. fresh coriander

Instructions:

- Mix the egg with a tablespoon of water. Warm the oil in a medium pan that doesn't stick. Add the egg and swirl it around the bottom of the pan like you're making a pancake. Cook until the egg is done. It doesn't need to be turned.

- Carefully flip the egg onto a board, spread it with salsa, sprinkle it with coriander, and then roll it up. It can be eaten hot or cold, and can be stored in the fridge for 2 days.

Nutritional values per serving: Calories 133 /kcal; Fat: 10 g; Carbs: 2 g; Fiber: 1 g; Protein: 9 g.

3.7 Kale Casserole With Mushrooms And Cheddar

Preparation time: 10 mins

Cooking time: 30 mins

Servings: 4

Ingredients:

- 2 large eggs

- 1 tbsp. melted butter, for greasing

- 2 tbsp. butter

- ¾ cup heavy whipping cream

- 3¼ cups mushrooms, sliced

- 2 garlic cloves, minced

- ¼ tsp. ground black pepper

- 1 tsp. salt

- 1 cup cream cheese

- 1 cup kale, trimmed and shredded

- 2 cups shredded cheddar cheese, divided

Instructions:

- Set oven temperature to 375°F. Grease a 9" x 9" using melted butter and keep it aside.

- Whisk the eggs and heavy whipping cream together in a small bowl. Set aside.

- In a large pan over medium heat, melt the butter. Add the mushrooms, garlic, salt, and pepper, and cook for a couple of minutes. The temperature should be raised to medium-high. Add the kale in small amounts and toss it for 5 minutes, or until it is soft.

- In the hot pan, mix the cream cheese with the fried vegetables. Mix in the egg mixture and half of the shredded cheddar cheese. Stir until everything is evenly mixed.

- Transfer the casserole mixture into the greased baking dish, and then sprinkle the rest of the cheddar cheese on top. Bake for about 20 to 25 minutes on the middle rack, or until the sides are golden brown and the middle is firm.

- Set aside for 10 minutes to cool down before serving.

Nutritional values per serving: Calories 125 /kcal; Fat: 12 g; Carbs: 4 g; Fiber: 2 g; Protein: 11 g.

3.8 Banana Bread

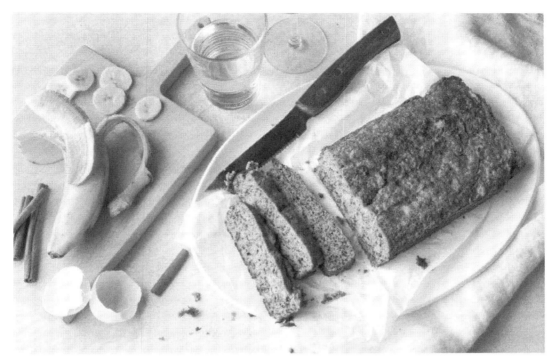

Preparation time: 15 mins

Cooking time: 50 mins

Servings: 12

Ingredients:

- 2 cups almond flour

- 1 tbsp. baking powder

- 1/4 cup coconut flour

- 1/2 tsp. xanthan gum

- 2 tsp. cinnamon

- 1/4 tsp. sea salt

- 2/3 cup fruit sweetener

- 1/2 cup unsalted butter, softened

- 1/2 cup unsweetened almond milk

- 4 large eggs, room temperature

- 1 cup chopped walnuts

- 2 tsp. banana extract

Instructions:

- Set the oven temperature to 350°F. Line and wrap parchment paper around in an 8.5-by-4.5-inch loaf pan so that it hangs over two opposite sides.

- Mix the coconut flour, almond flour, cinnamon, baking powder, xanthan gum, and sea salt together in a large bowl.

- In another large bowl, beat butter and sweetener with a hand mixer until fluffy.

- Beat in the eggs one at a time, then add the banana extract and almond milk.

- While the mixer is going at a medium speed, slowly add the dry ingredients to the wet ones until the mixture is thick and even.

- Add 3/4 cup of chopped walnuts and stir.

- Put the batter in the loaf pan, which has been lined, and press down evenly to make a smooth top. Sprinkle the rest of the chopped walnuts on top and lightly press them into the surface.

- Bake for 30–40 minutes, or until the top is golden. Cover the top with foil, and bake for another 20–25 minutes, or until a toothpick inserted into the center comes out clean.

- Let it cool all the way before taking it out of the pan and slicing it.

Nutritional values per serving: Calories 224 /kcal; Fat: 20 g; Carbs: 6 g; Fiber: 8 g; Protein: 4 g.

3.9 Vegetable Frittata

Preparation time: 10 mins

Cooking time: 20 mins

Servings: 8

Ingredients:

- 2 tbsp. olive oil

- 1 cup bell peppers, sliced

- 1 ½ cups mushrooms, sliced

- 8 large eggs

- 1 cup zucchini, cubed

- 3/4 tsp. sea salt

- 1/4 cup heavy cream

- 2/3 cup cheddar cheese, shredded

- 1/4 tsp. black pepper

Instructions:

- Set oven temperature to 375°F.

- On medium heat, heat the oil in a cast iron pan.

- Put in the veggies. Saute the vegetables for 6 to 10 minutes, stirring every so often, until they are soft and browned, and any extra water has evaporated.

- Mix the eggs, salt, cream, and pepper together in a large bowl with a whisk.

- Pour the egg and cream mixture into the pan and sprinkle the cheese on top. Mix them together slowly.

- Put the pan right away into an oven that has already been heated. Bake the frittata for about 15 to 20 minutes, until the surface is puffed up and the middle is just set. (Don't bake it too long or let it turn brown.) Take it out of the oven and let it rest for a few minutes before slicing it into pieces.

Nutritional values per serving: Calories 188 /kcal; Fat: 15 g; Carbs: 3 g; Fiber: 1 g; Protein: 11 g.

3.10 Breakfast Sandwich

Preparation time: 15 mins

Cooking time: 50 mins

Servings: 12

Ingredients:

- 2 cups blanched almond flour
- 2 tsp. baking powder
- ¼ cup sweetener
- 4 large eggs
- ½ tsp. maple extract
- ¼ tsp. sea salt
- 2/3 cup unsweetened almond milk
- 1 tsp. vanilla extract
- ¼ cup avocado oil

Egg layer:

- 1/8 tsp. black pepper
- 10 eggs
- ½ tsp. salt
- ½ cup unsweetened almond milk

Sausage layer:

- 1 tsp. maple extract
- 2 lb. breakfast sausage

Assembling:

- 2 cup cheddar cheese, shredded

Instructions:

- Set oven temperature to 425°F.

- Line two jelly-roll pans that are 15x10 inches with parchment paper and grease them properly.

- Mix all the pancake ingredients together in a large bowl with a whisk.

- Spread the batter out evenly in the pans that have been lined. Bake from both sides for 12 to 15 minutes, until golden and firm.

- Slip the parchment sheets off from the pancake layers and set them aside to cool.

- Don't change the oven's temperature. Put new sheets of parchment paper in both jelly-roll pans and grease them well.

Egg layer

- Put the egg mixture into one of the pans that has been lined.

- Bake the egg for about 15 minutes, or until it is firm and cooked all the way through.

- Slip the parchment sheets off from the egg layer and set it aside to cool. Don't change the oven's temperature.

Sausage layer

- Spread the sausage out in a thin layer on the second pan that has been lined with parchment paper. Press it as far as you can up the sides of the pan, because it will shrink as it cooks.

- Bake the sausage for 12 to 16 minutes, or until it is cooked all the way through. Drain the liquid and gently tap dry with paper towels.

- Don't turn off the oven, but turn it down to 350°F.

Assembling

- Use a large spatula to carefully slide between the pancake layers and the parchment paper. Repeat with the second layer of pancake, sausage and egg.

- Put a new sheet of parchment paper in one of the jelly-roll pans. Turn one of the pancake layers over so that the golden side is facing up.

- Put the sausage layer on top of the pancake layer, then put the egg layer on top of that, and then sprinkle the cheese on top evenly. The last step is to add the last pancake layer.

- Put the pan back in the oven for around 10 minutes, or till the cheese starts bubbling.

- After letting the pan rest for a few minutes, cut the sandwiches on the sheet pan into squares. Cut in a grid pattern: 3 across, 4 down, for a total of 12 sandwiches. You can eat the sandwiches right away, or you can let them cool to room temperature, wrap each one in foil or plastic wrap, put it in a freezer bag, and put it in the freezer.

Nutritional values per serving: Calories 541 /kcal; Fat: 46 g; Carbs: 5 g; Fiber: 2 g; Protein: 27 g.

3.11 Cauliflower Fritters

Preparation time: 10 mins

Cooking time: 20 mins

Servings: 3

Ingredients:

- ½ head cauliflower

- 1 tbsp. golden flax meal

- ½ cup scallions, thinly sliced

- 1 ½ tsp. salt

- 2 large eggs

- 3 tbsp. salted butter

- 1/2 tsp. pepper

- 3 tbsp. sour cream

Instructions:

- Grate the cauliflower and put it in a bowl. Add 1 tsp. salt and stir everything together well. Keep it at side for around 20 minutes.

- Put the cauliflower on a clean tea towel or a piece of muslin cloth. Press and squeeze out as much fluid as you can.

- Put the squeezed cauliflower in a clean bowl and add the rest of the ingredients, except the sour cream and butter. Blend well.

- Put the butter in a large nonstick pan and heat it over medium to high heat.

- When the pan is hot, add spoonful's of the prepared cauliflower mixture and flatten into small pancakes. Fry for 2–3 minutes on each side, until cooked properly and golden brown all the way through.

- Add a tablespoon of sour cream on each fritter and serve.

Nutritional values per serving: Calories 219 /kcal; Fat: 19 g; Carbs: 5 g; Fiber: 3 g; Protein: 8 g.

3.12 Savory Zucchini Muffins

Preparation time: 10 mins

Cooking time: 25 mins

Servings: 12

Ingredients:

- 12 oz. zucchini, grated

- ¼ tsp. salt

- ½ cup butter, melted

- 6 eggs

- ¼ tsp. pepper

- 1 cup cheddar cheese grated

- 1 tsp. baking powder

- 2 tbsp. oregano, finely chopped

- ¾ cup coconut flour

Instructions:

- Set oven temperature to 375°F.

- Put the zucchini, salt, melted butter, and pepper in a bowl and mix well.

- Mix well after adding the eggs, baking powder and oregano.

- Mix in the coconut flour until the batter thickens.

- Mix the cheddar cheese in with your hands. Use silicon cupcake molds to line a standard muffin tin, and the batter should be divided evenly between the muffin tins. If you put too much in each hole and make little piles of muffins, they don't rise very much.

- Bake the muffins for 25 minutes, or until they are golden brown.

- Give it 5 minutes to cool down before serving.

Nutritional values per serving: Calories 176 /kcal; Fat: 14 g; Carbs: 5 g; Fiber: 3 g; Protein: 7 g.

3.13 Carnivore Eggs

Preparation time: 10 mins

Cooking time: 10 mins

Servings: 4

Ingredients:

- 1 tbsp. salted butter

- 1 tsp. dried parsley

- 7 oz. ground beef

- ½ tsp. smoked paprika ground

- 1 tsp. cumin ground

- pepper to taste

- salt to taste

- 4 large eggs

- ½ cup cheddar cheese, shredded

Instructions:

- Set the oven temperature to 350°F.

- Put the butter in a pan that can go in the oven and heat it over high heat.

- Add the ground beef into the pan and sauté for one minute. After that add cumin, parsley and paprika in it and give it good mix.

- Season the beef mixture with salt and pepper to taste.

- Spread the meat mixture along the bottom of the skillet, and then make 4 holes for the eggs.

- Sprinkle the cheddar, and then break each egg into each hole.

- Take the pan off the heat and bake it for 5–10 minutes, or until the eggs are done the way you like.

- Serve right out of the pan or on a slice of toasted Keto Bread.

Nutritional values per serving: Calories 23 /kcal; Fat: 20 g; Carbs: 1.5 g; Fiber: 1 g; Protein: 19 g.

3.14 Spanish Baked Eggs

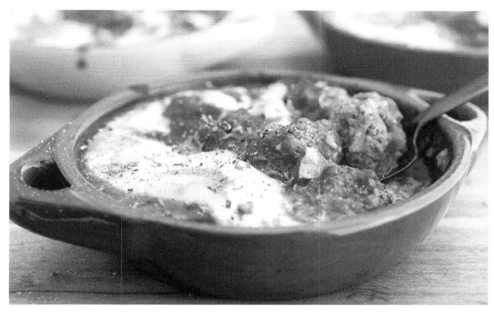

Preparation time: 10 mins

Cooking time: 18 mins

Servings: 2

Ingredients:

- 1 tbsp. olive oil

- 1/2 tsp. smoked paprika

- 1 smoked chorizo sausage, diced

- 1 tomato, diced

- 1/4 tsp. cumin ground

- 1 pinch salt

- 1/3 cup roasted peppers, strips

- 2 large eggs

- 1 pinch pepper

- 1 tsp. parsley, finely chopped

- 2 oz. manchego cheese, grated

Instructions:

- Preheat the oven to 390°F.

- Over medium heat, put the olive oil in a nonstick frying pan.

- Add the diced chorizo, cumin and paprika, and cook for 3–5 minutes, until the chorizo is cooked through.

- Add the diced tomatoes and keep cooking for about 5 minutes, or until the tomatoes are very soft.

- Now add the roasted peppers and season with salt and black pepper.

- Take the pan off the heat and divide the mixture into two dishes that are oven proof.

- Make a hole in the middle of the mixture, and crack one egg into each dish.

- Manchego cheese and parsley should be sprinkled on top.

- Put the dishes in the oven for 5 to 10 minutes, or until the egg is done the way you like it.

- Take the dish out of the oven and serve.

Nutritional values per serving: Calories 278 /kcal; Fat: 24 g; Carbs: 3 g; Fiber: 1 g; Protein: 12 g.

3.15 Breakfast Casserole

Preparation time: 10 mins

Cooking time: 50 mins

Servings: 8

Ingredients:

- 1 green bell pepper, diced

- 1/2 onion, diced

- 1 red pepper, diced

- 16 oz. mild breakfast sausage

- 2 cups fresh chopped spinach

- 1/2 cup half and half

- 12 eggs

- 1/2 tsp. salt

- 1/2 cup cheddar cheese, shredded

- 1/2 tsp. pepper

Instructions:

- Set the oven to 350°F and spray a casserole dish using cooking spray.

- Cook the sausage in a large pan over medium-high heat, breaking it up with a spatula as it cooks. Drain any extra grease released from the sausages and store the sausages in a separate container.

- Add all of the vegetables, excluding the spinach, to the same pan that was used to cook the sausage. Cook the vegetables for 4 minutes. When the vegetables are soft, add the spinach and cook for two more minutes. Put the sausage back in the pan with the vegetables and combine everything together. Take the pan off of the heat.

- The eggs should be cracked into a big bowl. Next, add the half-and-half, salt, cheese, and pepper. Beat the eggs and milk until they are well mixed.

- Spread the mixture of sausage and vegetables in the prepared casserole dish. Then, pour the egg mixture over the sausage and vegetables in an even layer. If you need to, use a spoon to make sure the eggs are spread out evenly.

- Bake the casserole for 30 to 35 minutes at 350 degrees. The top of the casserole should be a little bit brown and a little bit firm. Give the casserole about 5 minutes to cool down, and then serve and enjoy.

Nutritional values per serving: Calories 360 /kcal; Fat: 27 g; Carbs: 7 g; Fiber: 2 g; Protein: 24 g.

Chapter 4: Lunch Recipes

4.1 Blue Cheese Pork Medallions

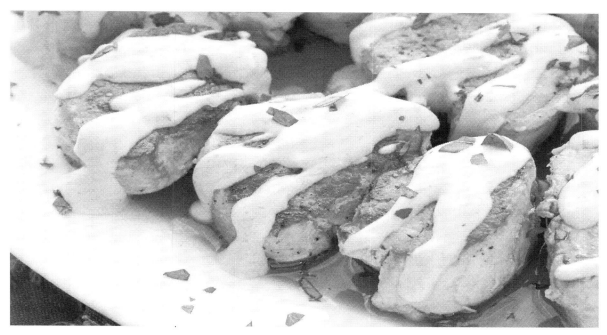

Preparation time: 15 mins

Cooking time: 10 mins

Servings: 4

Ingredients:

- 1 lb. tenderloin

- 2 tbsp. butter

- 2 tsp. Montreal steak seasoning

- ¼ cup crumbled blue cheese

- ½ cup heavy whipping cream

- 1 tbsp. fresh parsley, minced

Instructions:

- Slice the pork into 12 pieces and sprinkle steak seasoning on them. In a large skillet over medium heat melt the butter and a dd the pork, cover, and cook for 3–5 minutes per side, or until the meat is tender. Take the meat out from the pan and keep warm.

- Put the cream in the pan and bring it to a boil while stirring to loosen the bits from the pan. Cook for about 2 to 3 minutes, or until the cream is just a little bit thicker. Mix the cheese in until it melts. Serve this cream with pork and put some parsley on top as garnish.

Nutritional values per serving: Calories 317 /kcal; Fat: 23 g; Carbs: 1 g; Fiber: 0 g; Protein: 25 g.

4.2 Crockpot Curry Chicken

Preparation time: 25 mins

Cooking time: 6 hours

Servings: 4

Ingredients:

- 1.5 lbs. boneless chicken breast
- 15- oz. full-fat coconut milk
- 1 tbsp. minced garlic
- ½ tsp. garlic powder
- 3 tbsp. green curry paste
- ½ tsp. chili powder
- 1/8 tsp. salt
- 2 tbsp. fresh lime juice
- 2 tbsp. fresh Thai basil
- 1 large red pepper, sliced
- 1 large green pepper, sliced
- 1 tbsp. coconut oil
- ½ medium red onion, sliced
- 1/8 tsp. ground pepper

Instructions:

- Place the garlic powder, coconut milk, minced garlic, curry paste, salt, and chili powder into the slow cooker and stir everything together until combined.

- Soak the chicken breast in the gravy, trying to make sure that the chicken breasts are fully coated.

- Cover the slow cooker and continue to cook for 6 hours on low.

- When the chicken still has about 20 minutes to cook, get the onions and peppers ready.

- Heat coconut oil in a large pan over high heat.

- Then, add the sliced peppers and onions and sauté for about 5 minutes, just long enough to quickly fry them so they don't get soggy. Season the vegetables with salt and pepper. Take off the pan from the heat.

- When the chicken is fully cooked, take it out and shred it with two forks.

- Mix the sauce with the shredded chicken and put it back in the slow cooker. Add cooked peppers and onions, along with fresh lime juice and mix together.

- Serve with your favorite side and top with Thai basil.

Nutritional values per serving: Calories 455 /kcal; Fat: 26 g; Carbs: 8 g; Fiber: 2 g; Protein: 43 g.

4.3 Chicken Parmesan

Preparation time: 5 mins

Cooking time: 30 mins

Servings: 4

Ingredients:

- 4 chicken breast, thinly sliced

- ½ tsp. black pepper

- 1 cup mozzarella cheese, shredded

- 1 egg, beaten

- salt to taste

- 1/2 cup almond flour

- 1 cup Parmesan cheese, grated

- 1 tbsp. parsley

- 1 tsp. garlic powder

- 1 cup marinara sauce

- 2 tbsp. olive oil

Instructions:

- Preheat oven to 375°F. Spread a small amount of marinara sauce at the base of a large baking dish that has been sprayed using cooking spray. Use salt and pepper to season both sides of the chicken.

- Beat eggs in a small bowl. Mix the almond flour, grated parmesan, garlic powder, parsley, and onion powder in a separate medium bowl.

- Coat each chicken piece firstly in the egg and then in the grated parmesan mixture. Make sure every piece of chicken is completely covered.

- Put the olive oil in a pan and place it on medium-high heat. Lightly fry each piece of breaded chicken for about a minute on each side. Make sure the chicken doesn't lose its breading.

- Set each chicken piece in the baking dish. Put the same amount of marinara on each piece of chicken. Bake the parmesan chicken at 375°F for 20 minutes.

- Take the dish out of the oven and put the same amount of shredded mozzarella on each piece. Put the dish back in the oven and bake for another 10 to 15 minutes, or until the cheese is completely bubbly and melted. Take out of the oven and serve right away.

Nutritional values per serving: Calories 375 /kcal; Fat: 21 g; Carbs: 9 g; Fiber: 2 g; Protein: 37 g.

4.4 Thai Beef Curry

Preparation time: 15 mins

Cooking time: 50 mins

Servings: 6

Ingredients:

- 2 tbsp. coconut oil
- 2 lb. beef chuck diced 1in thick
- 3 kaffir lime leaves, shredded
- 16 oz. coconut milk
- salt to taste
- 2 tbsp. fish sauce
- ¼ cup peanuts crushed, for serving

Panang Paste

- 2 cloves garlic
- 2 scallions, roughly chopped
- ½ small onion, diced
- 1 lemongrass stalk white part only, sliced lengthwise
- 1/2- inch galangal, chopped
- 1 tbsp. cilantro, stems only
- 1-2 bird's eye chili
- 1 tsp. cumin
- 1 tsp. coriander
- ½ tsp. salt
- 1 tsp. shrimp paste

Instructions:

- Put all the ingredients of the panang paste into a food processor and blend them until they form a paste. If it doesn't blend well, you can add 1 tbsp. of water in the processor.

- Put the coconut oil in a wok or a pot and put it over high heat.

- Add the kaffir lime leaves for a minute and then add the prepared panang paste in the wok.

- After 5–7 minutes, add the beef and stir well.

- When the beef has been browned, add the rest of the ingredients, turn the heat down to low, partially cover the pot, and let it simmer for 30–45 minutes.

- Once the beef is soft and the sauce has separated from the oil and thickened, taste it and adjust the seasoning as needed.

- Serve with the peanuts on top and Keto Cauliflower Rice on the side.

Nutritional values per serving: Calories 509 /kcal; Fat: 41 g; Carbs: 5 g; Fiber: 2 g; Protein: 33 g.

4.5 Chicken Fajita Casserole

Preparation time: 10 mins

Cooking time: 50 mins

Servings: 12

Ingredients:

- 3 chicken breasts

- ½ onion, sliced

- 2 bell peppers, sliced

- 2 tbsp. taco seasoning, divided

- ¼ cup canned green chilies and tomatoes, diced

- 8 oz. cream cheese, softened

- 1 cup shredded cheese, divided

- ¼ cup heavy cream

Instructions:

- Set oven temperature to 350°F.

- Lightly season chicken using salt and pepper, and then bake them for 20 to 25 minutes in the preheated oven.

- While the chicken is in the oven, sauté the onion, bell peppers, diced tomatoes and green chiles in a skillet that has been greased. Cook the vegetables till they are soft, and then put them in a large bowl.

- Take the chicken out of the oven and let it cool for a while. Then, slice the chicken into pieces that are easy to eat and add them to the bowl with the onions and peppers.

- Use 1 tablespoon of taco seasoning to season the vegetables and chicken all over.

- In the bowl with the chicken and peppers, add all of the cream cheese, half of the shredded cheese, and the heavy cream. Blend everything together. Then, add the rest of the taco seasoning and stir again until everything is mixed well.

- Put the mixture in a casserole dish and sprinkle the rest of the shredded cheese on top. Bake for 30 to 35 minutes in an oven and serve piping hot.

Nutritional values per serving: Calories 191 /kcal; Fat: 7 g; Carbs: 6 g; Fiber: 1 g; Protein: 13 g.

4.6 Mexican Style Stuffed Peppers

Preparation time: 5 mins

Cooking time: 40 mins

Servings: 6

Ingredients:

- 3 bell peppers, halved

- ½ onion, chopped

- 1 lb. ground beef

- 1 cup rice cauliflower, steamed

- 2 cloves garlic, minced

- 1½ cups shredded cheese, divided

- 1 can chilies and tomatoes, diced

- 2½ tbsp. taco seasoning

Instructions:

- Set oven temperature to 400°F.

- Put a large pan over medium-high heat. Add garlic and onions in it and sauté for 2 minutes. Now add beef and keep cooking. Once the beef is done cooking, drain any extra grease and put it back in the pan.

- Turn the stove heat to medium. Mix the beef with the steamed cauliflower, chopped green chilies and tomatoes, and 1 cup of the shredded cheese. Add the taco seasoning to the mix and stir everything together.

- Put the pepper halves in a 9-by-13-inch baking dish. Then, put an equal amount of the beef filling into each pepper. Put the last 1/2 cup of cheese on top of each pepper in an even amount.

- Cover the peppers with foil in a loose way and bake them at 400°F for 30 minutes.

- Serve right away.

Nutritional values per serving: Calories 345 /kcal; Fat: 23 g; Carbs: 7 g; Fiber: 1 g; Protein: 28 g.

4.7 Spinach Stuffed Chicken Breast

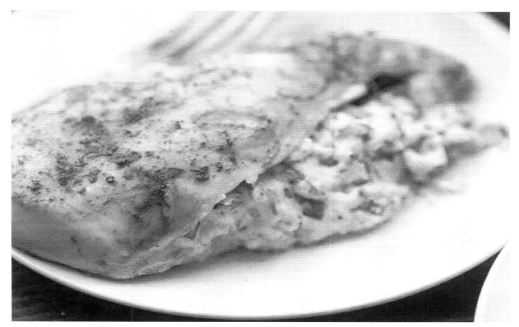

Preparation time: 10 minutes

Cooking time: 30 minutes

Servings: 4

Ingredients:

- 4 thick-cut chicken breast

- ½ tsp. garlic powder

- 1 tbsp. olive oil

- ½ tsp. paprika

- ½ tsp. onion powder

- 4 oz. cream cheese, softened

- salt and pepper, to taste

- 1 cup fresh spinach, chopped

- 1 cup mozzarella cheese, shredded

- ¼ tsp. garlic powder

Instructions:

- Preheat the oven to 375°F.

- Cut the chicken breasts from centre and create a pocket for filling.

- Rub olive oil all over the chicken, and then sprinkle onion powder, garlic powder, salt, paprika, and pepper on each side.

- Mix together the mozzarella, cream cheese, 1/4 teaspoon of garlic powder, spinach, salt, and pepper in a medium-sized bowl.

- Put the chicken breasts in an ovenproof dish.

- Stuff each piece of chicken breast pocket with the cheese mixture. Ensure that the filling goes deep into the chicken's pocket so it doesn't spill out while it's baking.

- Cover the chicken with foil and bake it for 25 to 30 minutes, or until it is fully cooked.

Nutritional values per serving: Calories 417 /kcal; Fat: 24 g; Carbs: 3 g; Fiber: 0 g; Protein: 46 g.

4.8 Chicken Bacon Ranch Casserole

Preparation time: 10 mins

Cooking time: 25 mins

Servings: 8

Ingredients:

- 5 cups broccoli florets

- 8 oz. cream cheese, softened

- 1 ½ lb. cooked chicken breast, cubed

- 1 cup cheddar cheese, shredded

- ¾ cup sour cream

- 1 packet ranch seasoning

- 1/2 cup crumbled bacon

- 1 cup Colby Jack cheese, shredded

Instructions:

- Set oven temperature to 350°F.

- Steam the broccoli. If you are using fresh broccoli, put it in a medium-sized bowl with half a cup of water. Wrap the bowl in cling film and heat it for 4 minutes in the microwave. If you are cooking with frozen broccoli, follow the directions on the package for how to cook it.

- In a large bowl, mix together the chicken, cream cheese, steamed broccoli, shredded cheddar, sour cream, and bacon. Mix everything properly.

- Now add the ranch seasoning combine everything again so that the seasoning is evenly spread.

- Spread the mixture into a 9x13-inch casserole dish and sprinkle the Colby Jack shredded cheese on top.

- Bake uncovered in the oven for 25 minutes, or until the cheese is melted.

- Crumble more bacon on top if you want, and enjoy.

Nutritional values per serving: Calories 444 /kcal; Fat: 28 g; Carbs: 9 g; Fiber: 2 g; Protein: 39 g.

4.9 Beef Stroganoff

Preparation time: 15 mins

Cooking time: 2 hours 20 minutes

Servings: 12

Ingredients:

- ¼ cup olive oil

- 2 cloves garlic, crushed

- 1 small onion, diced

- 3 lb. beef brisket, thinly sliced

- 2 tsp. dried thyme

- 1 tsp. salt

- ¼ cup tomato paste

- 1 tsp. pepper ground

- 2 cups beef stock

- ¼ cup red wine vinegar

- 1 cup sour cream

- 1 lb. mushrooms, sliced

Instructions:

- Put a large pot on high heat and a dd oil, garlic, onion and thyme in it.

- Saute the onion until it starts to become clear. Add the beef, pepper and salt and cook it until the beef turns brown.

- Now add the tomato paste and cook for 5 minutes. After five minutes now add the red wine vinegar in the pot and simmer it for the next 5 minutes.

- Add the beef stock and turn the heat down to low. Simmer for 1 hour with the lid off.

- Put in the mushrooms and keep cooking for another hour.

- Take the pot off the heat and mix in the sour cream.

- Taste it, and if you want, add more salt and pepper.

- Serve right away with Buttery Cauliflower Mash on the side.

Nutritional values per serving: Calories 482 /kcal; Fat: 38 g; Carbs: 3 g; Fiber: 1 g; Protein: 30 g.

4.10 Orange Chicken

Preparation time: 20 mins

Cooking time: 30 mins

Servings: 4

Ingredients:

- 1½ lb. boneless chicken breast, cubed

- 2 large eggs

- 1½ cups pork rind crumbs

- salt and pepper to taste

- 2 tbsp. heavy whipping cream

- 2 tsp. minced garlic

- oil for frying

- ½ tsp. sesame oil

- 1 tsp. ginger paste

- 2 tbsp. soy sauce

- 3 tbsp. water

- zest from one orange

- 1/3 cup brown sugar substitute

- ¼ cup white vinegar

- 2 tbsp. fresh orange juice

Instructions:

- Add oil in a large pan and heat it over medium-high heat.

- In a small bowl, mix the heavy cream and the eggs together.

- Dip the pieces of chicken in the egg mixture, and then roll them in the pork rind crumbs.

- Add the coated chicken in the pot and sprinkle salt and pepper to taste. Saute until it turns brown and is fully cooked.

- Take the chicken out and put it to the side.

- Put the minced garlic, sesame oil, ginger paste, soy sauce, water, orange zest, brown sugar substitute, white vinegar and fresh orange juice in a bowl and mix them together.

- Take out any extra oil from the pan and turn the heat down to medium.

- Pour the sauce mixture into the pot and let it cook until it thickens.

- Toss the chicken in the sauce and let it cool a bit before serving with chopped green onions and sesame seeds.

Nutritional values per serving: Calories 328/kcal; Fat: 13 g; Carbs: 2 g; Fiber: 1 g; Protein: 47 g.

4.11 Creamy Lemon Chicken

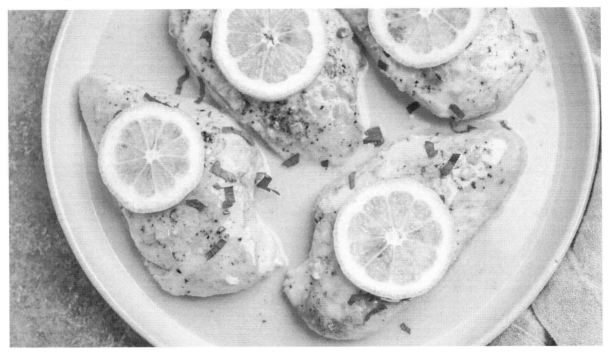

Preparation time: 10 mins

Cooking time: 28 mins

Servings: 6

Ingredients:

- 6 chicken thighs, boneless and skinless

- 1/2 tsp. garlic powder

- salt and pepper, to taste

- ¼ cup butter

- 1 tbsp. olive oil

- ½ cup chicken broth

- 3 cloves garlic, minced

- 1 tbsp. lemon juice

- 1 cup heavy cream

- 1 tbsp. arrowroot powder

- 1 lemon, sliced

Instructions:

- Marinate the chicken thighs using salt, garlic powder and pepper.

- Add the olive oil to a nonstick skillet and place it on on medium heat. Add the seasoned chicken to the pan and cook for about 7 minutes from each side, or until the temperature inside reaches 165°F.

- When the chicken is done cooking, take it out of the pan and set it aside.

- Put the minced garlic and butter in the same pan. Let the butter melt and cook the garlic for about a minute.

- As you stir, add the chicken broth and start scraping the brown bits off the bottom of the pan. Give the broth about 5 minutes to simmer.

- Mix the lemon juice and heavy cream and add it to the pan. Bring the sauce to a light boil, and then turn the heat down to medium. Give the sauce another 5 minutes to cook. For the sauce to be thicker, you can add arrowroot powder at this step.

- Put the chicken back in the pan and cook it for 3 more minutes. Add slices of lemon on top as a garnish and serve.

Nutritional values per serving: Calories 415 /kcal; Fat: 33 g; Carbs: 3 g; Fiber: 0 g; Protein: 29 g.

4.12 Crustless Ham And Swiss Quiche

Preparation time: 10 mins

Cooking time: 35 mins

Servings: 6

Ingredients:

- 5 Eggs

- ½ cup milk

- ½ cup heavy cream

- 8 oz. Swiss cheese, shredded

- 1 cup chopped ham

- 1 tsp. thyme

- 1 cup cubed zucchini

- ½ tsp. black pepper

- Salt to taste

- 2 tbsp. butter

Instructions:

- Turn oven on to 375°F.

- Melt 1 tbsp. of butter in a skillet over medium heat, add the chopped ham, and cook it until it's just a little bit browned.

- Take it out of the pan and put aside.

- Melt 1 tablespoon of butter in a pan and add zucchini in the pan. Cook until just a little bit soft.

- In a bowl, combine the eggs, milk, cream, salt, thyme, and pepper.

- Layer ham, ¾ part of the cheese, and zucchini in an 8- to 9-inch pan that has been greased lightly. Pour in the egg mixture and sprinkle the rest of the cheese on top.

- Bake in an oven that has been preheated for 35 to 40 minutes, or until a knife or toothpick stuck in the middle comes out clean.

Nutritional values per serving: Calories 361 /kcal; Fat: 30 g; Carbs: 4 g; Fiber: 0 g; Protein: 19 g.

4.13 Shepherd's Pie

Preparation time: 20 mins

Cooking time: 55 mins

Servings: 8

Ingredients:

Pie

- 2 tbsp. olive oil
- 2 cloves garlic, crushed
- 1 medium onion, diced
- 1 tsp. salt
- 1 tbsp. thyme fresh
- 3 large tomatoes, diced
- 2 lb. ground lamb
- 8 oz. lamb stock
- 1 medium zucchini, diced
- 7 oz. mushrooms, sliced

Mash

- 3 oz. butter
- 28 oz. cauliflower cut into florets
- 2 egg yolks
- 3.5 oz. cheddar cheese, shredded
- 1/2 tsp. pepper
- 1 tsp. salt

Topping

- 2.5 oz. cheddar cheese, shredded

Instructions:

Pie

- Place a large pot on the stove over medium-high heat.

- Add the oil, garlic, onion, thyme, and salt, and cook until the onion turns translucent. The ground lamb should be broken up and added to the pot at this point.

- With a wooden spoon, break up the meat into smaller chunks as it cooks and browns.

- When the meat is cooked through, add the chopped tomatoes and stock. Simmer this mixture for 20 minutes.

- Add the mushrooms and cook for 15 more minutes on low heat.

- Put in the zucchini, let it cook for 5 minutes, and then turn off the heat.

- Pour this lamb pie filling into your casserole dish and set it aside for a few minutes to cool down.

- Turn the oven on to 375°F.

Mash

- Fill a saucepan with 6 cups of water.

- Add the cauliflower and boil for about 10 minutes, or until it is soft.

- Drain the cauliflower properly and then return to the saucepan.

- Add butter into the cauliflower and blend the cauliflower into a puree form with the help of a stick blender.

- Add the cheese and mix until it melts and is evenly distributed.

- Add the salt and pepper and egg yolks and blend well.

- Spread the mashed cauliflower evenly on top of the Lamb Pie filling.

Topping

- Add cheddar cheese to the top of the cauliflower mash.

- Bake for 20 to 25 minutes or until the cheese turns brown.

- Take it out of the oven, serve it, and enjoy it!

Nutritional values per serving: Calories 568 /kcal; Fat: 47 g; Carbs: 8 g; Fiber: 2 g; Protein: 27 g.

4.14 Philly Cheesesteak Casserole

Preparation time: 10 mins

Cooking time: 40 mins

Servings: 5

Ingredients:

- 1 lb. shaved steak meat

- ½ cup green bell pepper, sliced

- 1 tsp. steak seasoning

- ½ cup onion, sliced

- ½ cup red bell pepper, sliced

- ¾ cup heavy whipping cream

- 2 tbsp. olive oil

- 1 cup Italian blend cheese, divided

- 3 oz. cream cheese

- freshly chopped parsley, for garnish

- salt and pepper to taste

Instructions:

- Set the oven temperature to 350°F.

- Put 1 tablespoon of olive oil and the thinly sliced steak in a pan over medium-high heat.

- Steak seasoning, salt, and pepper, to taste, should be sprinkled on the meat, which should then be sautéed until it is fully cooked. Take the meat out of the pan and set it aside.

- Add the last tablespoon of olive oil and the peppers and onions to the pan.

- Add salt and pepper to taste, and then cook the vegetables until they start to get soft.

- Add the cream cheese, heavy whipping cream, salt, and pepper to taste to a saucepan and heat it over medium heat. Keep cooking until the cream cheese melts and the sauce becomes thick.

- Mix together 1/2 cup of the shredded cheese and the sauce.

- Put the meat and vegetables in a 9x9 baking dish that has been well greased. Pour the sauce on top and toss to coat.

- Sprinkle the rest of the 1/2 cup cheese on top, and bake for 20 minutes, or till the cheese on top is bubbling and golden brown.

- Let it sit for a few minutes, sprinkle it with freshly chopped parsley, and serve.

Nutritional values per serving: Calories 526 /kcal; Fat: 45 g; Carbs: 5 g; Fiber: 1 g; Protein: 26 g.

4.15 Creamy Shrimp Alfredo With Zucchini Noodles

Preparation time: 15 mins

Cooking time: 15 mins

Servings: 5

Ingredients:

- 1 tbsp. garlic, minced

- ¼ cup unsalted butter

- ¼ tsp. pepper

- ¼ tsp. salt

- 1 cup heavy cream

- 1 lb. shrimp, peeled and deveined

- salt and pepper, to taste

- 1 cup Parmesan cheese, grated

- 1 cup spinach, chopped

- ¼ tsp. garlic powder

- 1 ½ lb. zucchini, spiralized

Instructions:

- Spread out zucchini noodles on a sheet of paper towels and lightly salt them. Leave them aside while you get the rest of the meal ready.

- Rinse the shrimp that have been peeled and deveined and pat them dry with paper towels. Add 1/4 teaspoon of salt and 1/4 teaspoon of pepper to the shrimps and then set them aside.

- Heat a large pan over medium-high heat to get it ready.

- Put the butter in the pan and allow it to melt.

- Add the garlic and seasoned shrimps once the butter has melted. Saute the shrimps for 2 minutes until they turn a light pink color. Make sure to stir the shrimp around in the pan so that they all cook at the same rate.

- When the shrimp are about halfway done, add the heavy cream to the pot and bring to a simmer. It's important to add the heavy cream before the shrimp are fully cooked, because once the cream is added, the shrimp will keep cooking. This will stop the shrimp from cooking too much.

- Once the sauce starts to simmer, add the Parmesan cheese in the pot and stir. Turn the heat down to medium and keep stirring until the sauce gets creamy.

- Add garlic powder, salt, and pepper to taste to the Alfredo sauce.

- Turn down the heat. Add the zucchini noodles and chopped spinach. Stir until the zucchini is warm all the way through.

- Take the pan off the heat and serve right away.

Nutritional values per serving: Calories 470 /kcal; Fat: 34 g; Carbs: 12 g; Fiber: 2 g; Protein: 31 g.

Chapter 5: Dinner Recipes

5.1 Creamy Tuscan Chicken

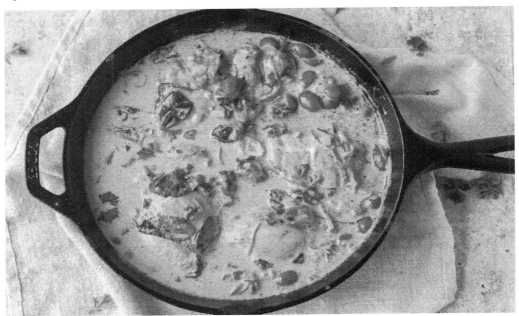

Preparation time: 10 mins

Cooking time: 25 mins

Servings: 6

Ingredients:

- 2 tbsp. olive oil

- 3 garlic cloves, minced

- 2 ¼ lb. boneless, skinless chicken breasts

- 1/2 tsp. paprika

- 1/2 tsp. Italian seasoning

- 2 tbsp. butter

- 1/2 cup chicken broth

- 1/2 cup Parmesan cheese, freshly grated

- 1/4 onion, chopped

- 1 ¼ cup heavy whipping cream

- 1 cup grape tomatoes. halved

- 1/3 cup Gouda cheese, freshly grated

- 1 ½ cup baby spinach leaves, chopped

Instructions:

- Season the chicken breasts using salt, pepper, and Italian seasoning.

- Add 2 tablespoons of olive oil to a 12-inch cast-iron pan and set it over medium heat.

- When the pan is hot, add the chicken and sear it until brown on both sides. Cover the chicken with a lid to help it cook. Don't cook the chicken for too long. The temperature inside should be 165°F.

- Add garlic, butter, onion, diced tomatoes, and paprika to the pan. Cook on medium/low heat for 5 minutes, stirring every so often.

- Use chicken broth to clean the pan. Scrape the bottom of the pan to get rid of any food that might have stuck there. Keep them in the pan, because they add a lot of flavor.

- Add Parmesan cheese, heavy cream, Gouda, and spinach. Simmer on medium heat until the sauce starts to thicken, stirring every so often so it doesn't stick.

- Put the chicken back in the pan and let it cook for two minutes on low heat.

Nutritional values per serving: Calories 524 /kcal; Fat: 37 g; Carbs: 4 g; Fiber: 1 g; Protein: 44 g.

5.2 Chicken Parmesan Casserole

Preparation time: 5 mins

Cooking time: 40 mins

Servings: 8

Ingredients:

- 2 cups shredded mozzarella cheese

- 4 chicken breasts, cubed

- 2 cups Marinara Sauce

- ½ cup ground pork rinds, plain

- 1 cup almond flour

- 2 tsp. garlic powder

- 1 ¼ cups grated parmesan cheese, divided

- ½ tsp. dried basil

- 1 tbsp. dried parsley

- ¼ tsp. fresh ground pepper

- ¼ tsp. oregano

- 2 eggs, beaten

- ½ tsp. salt

- Olive oil for frying

Instructions:

- Turn the oven on to 400°F.

- Use a food processor or mini-chopper to chop up the pork rinds. Take out and put away. Add cubes of Parmesan cheese into the food processor and process until the mixture has a texture like pork rinds.

- Put all of the dry ingredients, except for 1/4 cup of the grated parmesan cheese, in a bowl and mix with a whisk or fork until everything is well blended.

- Place beaten eggs, chicken, and breading mixture on the counter shelf. Coat the chicken pieces one by one in the egg and then in the breading mixture.

- Heat a large skillet over medium-high heat, then fry the chicken for several minutes on each side in a little bit of olive oil. They don't have to be cooked all the way through because the oven will finish cooking them. Take it out and let it drain on some paper towels. Put the nuggets in a big bowl to mix. Mix in 1 cup of the shredded mozzarella cheese with the marinara sauce.

- Pour the mixture into a nonstick-sprayed 9" x 13" glass baking dish. Put 1 cup of mozzarella cheese and the reserved 1/4 cup of grated parmesan cheese on top, then bake for 25 minutes or till the cheese is golden brown.

- Let it cool down a bit before serving.

Nutritional values per serving: Calories 389 /kcal; Fat: 20 g; Carbs: 8 g; Fiber: 4 g; Protein: 39 g.

5.3 Shrimp Scampi With Zucchini Noodles

Preparation time: 12 mins

Cooking time: 13 mins

Servings: 4

Ingredients:

- 2 tbsp. olive oil

- 1/2 tsp. sea salt

- 1 lb. large shrimps

- 1 tbsp. olive oil

- 1/4 tsp. black pepper

- 1 medium shallot, minced

- 4 cloves garlic, minced

- 1/4 cup unsalted butter

- 1/4 cup parsley, chopped

- 1/4 cup chicken bone broth

- 1/2 tsp. sea salt

- 2 tbsp. lemon juice

- 1 lb. zucchini, spiralized

- 1/4 tsp. black pepper

Instructions:

- Add salt to the zucchini noodles and put them in a colander over the sink. Leave them for 20 minutes. The salt will make the water come out.

- In a large sauté pan, heat 2 tablespoons of oil over medium-high heat.

- Add in the shrimp. Add salt and pepper according to your taste. Arrange everything in one layer. Saute for 2 to 3 minutes without moving, till the corners start to turn clear and the bottom starts to brown. Turn the shrimps over and cook for 1–3 more minutes, or until it's done. Take the shrimp out of the pan and cover it to keep it warm.

- Put in another tablespoon of oil. Add the garlic and shallots that have been chopped to the pan. Saute for about 2–3 minutes, until the food turns brown.

- Deglaze the pan by adding broth and scraping the bottom. Simmer for 2 to 3 minutes, or until half of the liquid is gone.

- Add lemon juice and butter and stir. After the butter melts, bring to a simmer and cook for 3–4 more minutes, mixing occasionally and scraping the base of the pan, until the volume is reduced. Season it with a pinch of salt and pepper and add chopped parsley.

- Once the zucchini seems soft and watery, gently squeeze the zoodles to get some more water out. Don't try to squeeze hard to get every last drop, or the noodles will get mushy. Add the noodles made from zucchini to the pan. Cook for 2-3 minutes, just until hot.

- Put the shrimp back in the pan and stir it. Serve and enjoy.

Nutritional values per serving: Calories 341 /kcal; Fat: 24 g; Carbs: 6 g; Fiber: 2 g; Protein: 26 g.

5.4 Chipotle Beef Barbacoa

Preparation time: 10 mins

Cooking time: 4 hours

Servings: 12

Ingredients:

- 3 lb. Beef brisket, chunks

- 2 medium Chipotle chiles in adobo

- 1/2 cup Beef broth

- 2 tbsp. Apple cider vinegar

- 5 cloves Garlic, minced

- 1 tbsp. Dried oregano

- 2 tbsp. Lime juice

- 2 tsp. Sea salt

- 2 tsp. Cumin

- 1/2 tsp. Ground cloves, optional

- 1 tsp. Black pepper

- 2 whole Bay leaves

Instructions:

- In a blender, mix the chipotle chiles in adobo sauce, broth, apple cider vinegar, garlic, dried oregano, lime juice, sea salt, cumin, black pepper, and ground cloves. Blend until it's smooth.

- Put the chunks of beef in the slow cooker. Pour the mixture that from the blender on top. Add the bay leaves in the pot and cook on high for 4 hours, until the beef is juicy and soft.

- Take the bay leaves away. With two forks, shred the meat and mix it into the juices. Cover the beef and let it sit for 5–10 minutes so that it can soak up even more flavor. To serve, use a slotted spoon.

Nutritional values per serving: Calories 213 /kcal; Fat: 13 g; Carbs: 2 g; Fiber: 0.6 g; Protein: 22 g.

5.5 Eggplant Lasagna

Preparation time: 20 mins

Cooking time: 40 mins

Servings: 8

Ingredients:

- 20 oz. eggplant, sliced lengthwise into 8 slices

- 1/4 tsp. black pepper

- 1/4 tsp. sea salt

- 2 tbsp. olive oil

Meat sauce

- 2 cloves garlic, minced

- 1 tsp. olive oil

- 1 tsp. sea salt

- 1 ½ lb. ground beef

- 1 ½ cups marinara sauce

- 1/2 tsp. black pepper

- 1 tbsp. Italian seasoning

Cheese topping

- 2 cups mozzarella cheese

Cheese filling

- 8 oz. ricotta cheese

- 1 large egg

- 1/2 cup grated parmesan cheese

Instructions:

- Set the oven temperature to 400°F. Line a baking sheet and grease it.

- Place the slices of eggplant in a single layer on a greased baking sheet. Season the eggplant slices with salt and pepper and brush o live oil on both sides of eggplant slices.

- For about 15–25 minutes, or until soft, roast the eggplant in the oven. When the slices are roasted, take them out of the oven but keep the oven switched on.

- Heat oil at medium temperature in a large pan. Add the garlic in the pan and fry for about a minute, or until the garlic smells good.

- Turn the heat up to high and add the ground beef. Add sea salt and black pepper to taste. Cook until the meat is browned, about 10 minutes. Use a spoon or spatula to break up the meat as it cooks.

- Season the beef with Italian seasoning and Marinara sauce should be stirred in. Turn down the heat to a slow simmer. For about 10 minutes, let it simmer.

- Make the cheese filling while the meat sauce is cooking. Mix the Parmesan cheese, ricotta cheese, and egg in a small bowl.

- Layer roasted eggplant slices in a single layer on the bottom of casserole dish. Put the ground beef and marinara sauce mixture on top. The ricotta mixture should be spread on top. Shred some mozzarella cheese and sprinkle it on top. Do it again, ending with the shredded mozzarella.

- Bake for 10–15 minutes, or until the cheese on top is golden and bubbling.

Nutritional values per serving: Calories 426 /kcal; Fat: 30 g; Carbs: 6 g; Fiber: 3 g; Protein: 30 g.

5.6 Steak And Shrimp

Preparation time: 10 mins

Cooking time: 15 mins

Servings: 4

Ingredients:

- 1/2 tsp. fresh parsley, chopped

- 6 tbsp. unsalted butter, softened

- 1/2 tbsp. fresh rosemary, chopped

- 2 cloves garlic, minced

- 1/2 tbsp. fresh thyme

Shrimp

- 12 oz. medium shrimp

Steaks

- 1/2 tbsp. sea salt

- 1 tbsp. olive oil

- 1/2 tsp. black pepper

- 4 sirloin steaks, 1 inch thick

Instructions:

- Mix the garlic, butter, rosemary, thyme, and parsley together in a small bowl. Keep the garlic butter in the refrigerator until you are ready to use it.

- Take the steaks from the refrigerator 30 minutes before you cook them so that they can come to room temperature.

- Olive oil should be used to brush steaks from both sides. Salt and pepper both sides a lot, and pat to help the salt and pepper stick.

- Heat a cast iron grill pan for two to three minutes over medium-high heat, until it is very hot.

- Add the steaks and grill for 4 to 5 minutes, until the bottoms are browned. Flip and cook for another 2–7 minutes, or until it's done the way you like.

- Take the steaks out of the skillet. Cover them and leave them to rest and stay warm.

- Turn off the heat and wait until the pan stops smoking, and then clean it down carefully if there are any bits left.

- Even though the heat is off, the pan should still be hot, so add 2 tbsp. of garlic butter in small pieces. (Reserve the remaining garlic butter for serving the steaks.) Move the pieces of butter around as they melt so that the butter evenly covers the pan.

- Turn the heat up to medium once the butter has melted. Add the shrimp quickly in one layer. Saute for 1-3 minutes on each side, until colorless and golden.

- Put a pat of garlic butter on top of steaks to serve. Serve shrimp with the steaks. If you want, you can pour garlic butter from the pan over the shrimp and squeeze some lemon on top.

Nutritional values per serving: Calories 594 /kcal; Fat: 40 g; Carbs: 1 g; Fiber: 0.2 g; Protein: 52.8 g.

5.7 Crustless Zucchini Quiche

Preparation time: 10 mins

Cooking time: 40 mins

Servings: 6

Ingredients:

- 2 tbsp. olive oil

- 2 medium zucchini, sliced thinly

- 1/2 medium onion, diced

- 2 tsp. dried basil

- 7 large eggs

- 1/2 tsp. sea salt

- 4 cloves garlic, minced

- 1/3 cup cheddar cheese

- 1/3 cup heavy cream

- 1/4 tsp. black pepper

- 1/3 cup mozzarella cheese

Instructions:

- Set the oven temperature to 350°F.

- In a large pan over medium heat, heat the oil. Add in the onions and sauté for about 5 minutes, until they turn translucent.

- Slice the zucchini and sprinkle dried basil on top.

- Raise the temperature to medium-high. Add the zucchini, stirring every once in a while, for about 5 minutes, until it is tender and starting to brown.

- In the middle, make a well and add the minced garlic. Saute for about a minute, until the smell is nice, and then mix the garlic into the onions and zucchini.

- Put half of the zucchini mixture in the bottom of a 9-inch (23 cm) round pie pan or an 8-inch square baking pan. Cover the zucchini with half of each cheese. Add the rest of the zucchini and the rest of the cheeses on top.

- Whisk the cream, eggs, sea salt, and black pepper together in a large bowl. Pour the egg mix over the zucchini in the pan.

- Bake the quiche for 30-35 minutes, until firm.

Nutritional values per serving: Calories 229 /kcal; Fat: 18 g; Carbs: 5 g; Fiber: 1 g; Protein: 12 g.

5.8 Beef Stew

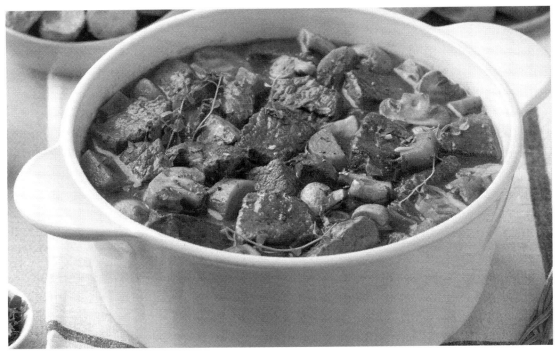

Preparation time: 15 mins

Cooking time: 1 hour

Servings: 6

Ingredients:

- 2 lb. beef chuck roast, cubed

- Freshly ground black pepper, to taste

- Kosher salt, to taste

- 8 oz. Baby bella mushrooms, sliced

- 2 tbsp. extra-virgin olive oil

- 1 medium carrot, sliced

- 1 small onion, chopped

- 3 cloves garlic, minced

- 2 stalks celery, sliced

- 1 tbsp. tomato paste

- 1 tsp. fresh thyme leaves

- 6 cups low-sodium beef broth

- 1 tsp. fresh rosemary, chopped

Instructions:

- Use paper towels to dry the beef, and then season it well with pepper and salt. Heat oil in a large pot over medium heat. Adding the beef one piece at a time, sear it on all sides until light golden, about 3 minutes on each side. Take the meat out of the pot and repeat the procedure with the rest of the meat, adding more oil if required.

- Add mushrooms to the same pot and cook for 5 minutes, until they are golden and crispy. Put in the carrots, onion, and celery, and cook for 5 minutes, until they are soft. Add the garlic and cook for another minute, until it smells good. Now add tomato paste and stir to coat the vegetables with tomato paste.

- Add broth, thyme, beef, rosemary, and salt and pepper to the pot. Bring to a boil, and then turn down the heat to a slow boil. Simmer for 45 minutes, or until the beef is soft.

Nutritional values per serving: Calories 280 /kcal; Fat: 13 g; Carbs: 8 g; Fiber: 1 g; Protein: 35 g.

5.9 Turkey Pie

Preparation time: 10 mins

Cooking time: 40 mins

Servings: 6

Ingredients:

Filling

- 1 cup turkey meat, cooked and shredded
- Salt to taste
- 2 cups turkey stock
- ½ tsp. black pepper
- ½ cup kale, chopped
- 1 tsp. thyme, chopped
- ½ cup cheddar cheese, shredded
- ½ cup butternut squash, peeled and chopped
- ¼ tsp. garlic powder
- ¼ tsp. paprika
- Cooking spray
- ¼ tsp. xanthan gum

Crust

- ¼ cup ghee
- A pinch of salt
- ¼ tsp. xanthan gum
- 2 cups almond flour
- ¼ cup cheddar cheese
- 1 egg

Instructions:

Filling

- Put the stock in a pot and heat it over medium heat.

- Stir in the turkey meat and squash, cook for 10 minutes and then a dd kale, garlic powder, paprika, thyme, salt, pepper, and 1/2 cup of the cheddar cheese.

- Mix 1/4 teaspoon of xanthan gum with 1/2 cup of stock from the pot in a bowl, stir well, and then add everything to the pot.

- Turn off the heat and put the pot at the side.

Crust

- Stir 1/4 teaspoon of xanthan gum and a pinch of salt into the flour in a bowl.

- Mix in the egg, ghee, and 1/4 cup of cheddar cheese until you get the dough for your pie crust.

- Form it into a ball and put it in the refrigerator for now.

Assembling

- Spread pie filling on the bottom of a baking dish that has been sprayed with cooking spray.

- Put the dough on a work surface, roll it into a circle, and put this on top of the filling.

- Press the dough well and seal the edges. Put it in the oven at 350°F for 35 minutes.

- Let the pie cool for a while and then serve.

Nutritional values per serving: Calories 320 /kcal; Fat: 23 g; Carbs: 6 g; Fiber: 8 g; Protein: 16 g.

5.10 Moroccan Meatballs

Preparation time: 20 mins

Cooking time: 5 hours

Servings: 8

Ingredients:

- 2 lb. ground beef

- 4 cloves garlic, crushed

- 1 small onion, grated

- 2 tbsp. cilantro, finely chopped

- 1 large egg

- 1 tbsp. coriander

- 1 tbsp. cumin

- 2 tsp. ground ginger

- 1 tbsp. smoked paprika

- 1 tsp. salt

- 1 tsp. cinnamon

- 2 tbsp. tomato paste

- 2 tbsp. olive oil

- ½ cup beef stock

- 1 ½ cups tomato puree

- 1/3 cup cilantro, for serving

Instructions:

- Mix the beef, half of the grated garlic, half of the grated onion, egg, cumin, cilantro, coriander, ginger, paprika, cinnamon, and salt together in a large bowl. Blend well.

- Roll into meatballs about the size of 2 tablespoons and set aside. This mixture will yield around 40 meatballs.

- Over high heat, place a non-stick frying pan and add oil, the rest of the garlic and onion and sauté for 3-5 minutes, until fragrant.

- Add the tomato paste and cook for another 3 minutes. Next, add the tomato puree and stock to your slow cooker. Blend well.

- Now add prepared meatballs in the sauce and cook for 5 hours on low heat.

- Mix in the cilantro, and serve with Cauliflower Mash on the side.

Nutritional values per serving: Calories 363/kcal; Fat: 27 g; Carbs: 5 g; Fiber: 2 g; Protein:

22 g.

5.11 Cheeseburger Casserole

Preparation time: 10 mins

Cooking time: 40 mins

Servings: 6

Ingredients:

- 1 tsp. olive oil

- ½ tsp. salt

- 1 lb. ground beef

- 5 oz. bacon diced

- ¼ tsp. white pepper ground

- 2 dill pickles, sliced

- 1 small onion, diced

- ¼ cup yellow mustard

- ¼ cup tomato ketchup, sugar-free

- 2 tbsp. Worcestershire sauce

- ¼ cup low carb mayonnaise

- 1 tsp. garlic powder

- 3 large eggs

- 1 cup cheddar cheese, shredded

- 1/4 cup heavy cream

Instructions:

- Set the oven's temperature to 375°F.

- Put a large pot on high heat and add the ground beef, oil, salt, and pepper in it. Break up the beef and cook it until it turns brown. Then, take the pot off the heat.

- Put the bacon in non-stick pan and cook it over high heat until it's crispy. Then, drain the fat and add the crispy fried bacon to the beef mixture.

- Mix the beef with the onion, ketchup, pickles, mayonnaise, mustard, Worcestershire sauce, garlic powder, and half of the cheese. Mix it well.

- The beef mixture should be put in a casserole dish.

- Whisk the eggs and cream together in a bowl, and then pour it over the beef mixture.

- Bake the casserole for 30 minutes with the rest of the cheese on top.

- Serve piping hot and enjoy.

Nutritional values per serving: Calories 534 /kcal; Fat: 45 g; Carbs: 5 g; Fiber: 1 g; Protein: 25 g.

5.12 Lamb Korma

Preparation time: 15 mins

Cooking time: 2 hours

Servings: 15

Ingredients:

- 4 lb. lamb shoulder, diced

- 6 cloves garlic

- 1 inch ginger

- 3 oz. ghee

- 1 small onion

- 2 tbsp. garam masala

- 1 cinnamon stick

- 1½ tbsp. coriander ground

- 1½ tbsp. ginger ground

- 1½ tbsp. cumin ground

- 2 tsp. turmeric ground

- 2 tsp. Kashmiri chili powder

- 1 cup water

- 1 cup heavy cream

- 1 tsp. white pepper

- 1-2 tsp. salt

- 11 oz. Greek yogurt

Instructions:

- Put the garlic, ginger, and onion in the food processor and pulse until the ingredients are very finely chopped.

- Put the ground ginger, garam masala, cumin, coriander, Kashmiri chili, and turmeric in a small bowl and mix them all together.

- Put the ghee in a large saucepan and heat it over low heat.

- Add the onion mixture and the cinnamon stick, and cook over low heat for 10 to 15 minutes, until the onions are clear and start turning brown.

- Turn the heat up to medium and add the lamb pieces. Cook until it turns brown.

- Stir the lamb to coat it with the spice mix.

- Add the cream and water, stir well, and bring the pot to a simmer.

- Turn the heat down to low and cover the pan halfway. Simmer for 2 hours, stirring after 20 minutes. The sauce will get just thick enough to cover the meat. If the pan is getting too dry, add half a cup more of water.

- Mix well after adding the pepper, salt and yogurt. Keep simmering for another 10 minutes, and then turn off the heat.

- Serve with a side of your choice and enjoy.

Nutritional values per serving: Calories 446 /kcal; Fat: 38 g; Carbs: 3 g; Fiber: 1 g; Protein: 23 g.

5.13 Lemon Butter Baked Tilapia

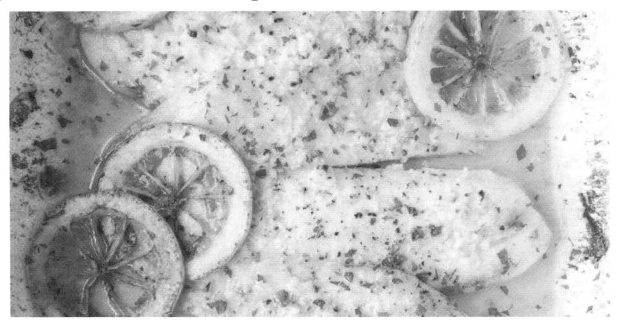

Preparation time: B10 mins

Cooking time: 15 mins

Servings: 4

Ingredients:

- 4 tilapia fillets

- 1 medium lemon

- ¼ cup unsalted butter

- 1 tsp. sea salt

- 2 cloves garlic, crushed

- 1 tbsp. fresh parsley

- ¼ tsp. black pepper

Instructions:

- Set the oven temperature to 400°F.

- Dry the fish fillets with paper towels. Put them in a 9x13 baking dish in a single layer.

- Cut lemon in half and juice and zest one half of the lemon. You will get 1/2 tbsp. of lemon zest and 1 tbsp. of lemon juice from one half. The other half should be cut into thin slices.

- Melt the butter in a small bowl in the microwave or in a saucepan on the stove. Mix in the lemon zest, parsley, lemon juice, and garlic into the melted butter.

- The fillets of tilapia should be covered with the garlic lemon butter. Add black pepper and sea salt to taste. Flip it over and apply the lemon butter and seasoning again. Put the slices of lemon on top of the fish.

- Bake the tilapia for 15 minutes or until its opaque and the fish flakes easily with a fork.

Nutritional values per serving: Calories 270 /kcal; Fat: 14 g; Carbs: 1 g; Fiber: 0.1 g; Protein: 34 g.

5.14 Blackened Tilapia With Zucchini Noodles

Preparation time: 20 mins

Cooking time: 10 mins

Servings: 4

Ingredients:

- 2 large zucchini

- ¾ tsp. salt, divided

- 1½ tsp. ground cumin

- ½ tsp. pepper

- ½ tsp. smoked paprika

- 2 garlic cloves, minced

- 4 tilapia fillets

- ¼ tsp. garlic powder

- 2 tsp. olive oil

- 1 cup pico de gallo, for serving

Instructions:

- Cut the ends of the zucchinis. Use a spiralizer to make thin strands of zucchini.

- Mix the cumin, 1/2 tsp. salt, pepper, smoked paprika and garlic powder together. Sprinkle this mixture generously on both sides of the tilapia. On medium-high heat, heat oil in a large nonstick pan. Cook the tilapia in batches for about 2-3 minutes per side, or until the fish just starts to flake apart easily with a fork. Take from the pan and keep warm.

- In the same pan, cook the zucchini noodles and garlic over medium-high heat for 1-2 minutes, tossing them around with tongs the whole time. Add the rest of the salt. Serve the noodles with fish and pico de gallo.

Nutritional values per serving: Calories 203 /kcal; Fat: 4 g; Carbs: 8 g; Fiber: 2 g; Protein: 34 g.

5.15 Creamy Dijon Chicken

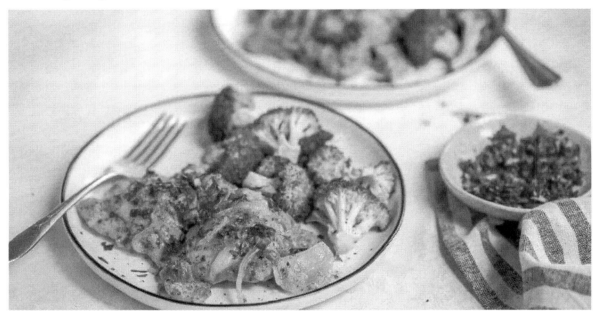

Preparation time: 10 mins

Cooking time: 15 mins

Servings: 4

Ingredients:

- ½ cup half-and-half cream

- 1 tbsp. brown sugar

- ¼ cup Dijon mustard

- 4 boneless chicken breast halves

- 2 tsp. olive oil

- ¼ tsp. pepper

- ¼ tsp. salt

- 1 small onion, thinly sliced

- 2 tsp. butter

- Minced fresh parsley, for garnish

Instructions:

- Mix mustard, cream, and brown sugar with a whisk. Use a meat mallet to even out the thickness of the chicken breasts, and then sprinkle them with salt and pepper.

- Over medium-high heat, melt the butter and oil in a large skillet. Brown the chicken from both sides. Turn heat down to medium. Bring to a boil, and then add the onion and cream mixture. Turn down the heat and simmer, covered, for 10–12 minutes, or until a thermometer inserted into the chicken reads 165°. Put some parsley on top and serve.

Nutritional values per serving: Calories 295 /kcal; Fat: 11 g; Carbs: 6 g; Fiber: 0 g; Protein: 36 g.

Chapter 6: Sides And Snacks

6.1 Buttery Cauliflower Mash

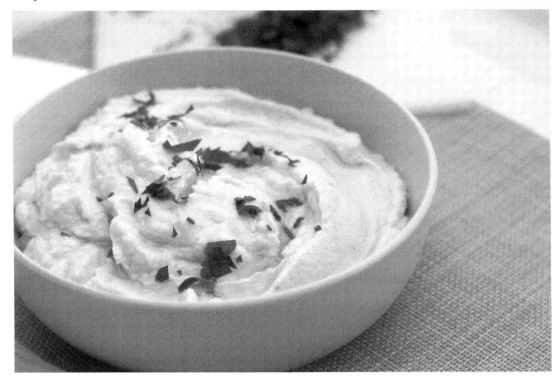

Preparation time: 10 mins

Cooking time: 10 mins

Servings: 5

Ingredients:

- 3 oz. butter

- 1 medium cauliflower

- ½ tsp. pepper

- 1 tsp. salt

Instructions:

- Bring water to boil in a large pot.

- Cut the cauliflower into florets of the same size.

- Add the cauliflower gently to the boiling water and boil for 5 to 8 minutes or until the cauliflower is soft.

- Drain the cauliflower really well, and then put it back in the pot that is still warm.

- Add the salt and pepper and the butter.

- Use a stick blender to mix the cauliflower until there are no more lumps.

- Let the mixture rest for 3 minutes, and then blend it again. This step of letting the cauliflower sit and then blending it makes it extra creamy and smooth.

- Serve with a main dish of your choice and enjoy.

Nutritional values per serving: Calories 151 /kcal; Fat: 14 g; Carbs: 6 g; Fiber: 3 g; Protein: 2 g.

6.2 Garlic Butter Mushrooms

Preparation time: 10 mins

Cooking time: 15 mins

Servings: 2

Ingredients:

- 1 tbsp. olive oil

- 1 tsp. sea salt flakes

- 4 cloves garlic, finely chopped

- 1 lb. button mushrooms

- ¼ tsp. pepper ground

- 2 tbsp. parsley, chopped

- 3 tbsp. butter

Instructions:

- Place a non-stick pan on high heat.

- Add the oil, garlic, salt, and pepper, and cook until the garlic smells good.

- Put the mushrooms in the pan coat them.

- Stir the mushrooms while adding the butter one tablespoon at a time. Let each tablespoon melt and coat the mushrooms before adding the next.

- Once the mushrooms start to give off liquid, turn the heat down to medium and stir every so often until all the liquid is gone and the mushrooms are a deep brown color.

- Take the pan off the heat and garnish with the parsley before you serve the mushrooms.

Nutritional values per serving: Calories 273 /kcal; Fat: 25 g; Carbs: 8 g; Fiber: 3 g; Protein: 8 g.

6.3 Keto Mac And Cheese

Preparation time: 20 mins

Cooking time: 1 hour

Servings: 8

Ingredients:

- Butter, for greasing dish

- 2 tbsp. extra-virgin olive oil

- 2 medium heads cauliflower, florets

- 1 cup heavy cream

- Kosher salt, to taste

- 4 cup shredded cheddar

- 6 oz. cream cheese, cubed

- 1 tbsp. hot sauce

- 2 cup shredded mozzarella

- 4 oz. pork rinds, crushed

- Freshly ground black pepper, to taste

- 1 tbsp. extra-virgin olive oil

- 1/4 cup freshly grated Parmesan

- 2 tbsp. fresh parsley, chopped

Instructions:

- Butter a 9"-x-13" baking dish and preheat the oven to 375°. Mix cauliflower with 2 tbsp. of oil and salt in a large bowl. Spread the cauliflower out on baking sheet and roast it for about 40 minutes, or until it is soft and lightly golden.

- While cauliflower is roasting, heat cream in a large pot over medium heat. Bring to a boil, and then turn the heat down to low and stir in the cheeses until they melt. Take the pan off the heat, add hot sauce, and season with salt and pepper. Stir in the roasted cauliflower. Taste and add more seasoning if necessary.

- Move mixture to a baking dish that has been prepared. In a medium bowl, mix the Parmesan, pork rinds, and oil together with a spoon. Spread the mixture on top of the cauliflower and cheese in an even layer.

- Bake until golden and crisp for about 15 minutes. If you want to toast the topping even more, turn the oven to broil for about 2 minutes.

- Add some parsley as a garnish before serving.

Nutritional values per serving: Calories 665 /kcal; Fat: 55 g; Carbs: 12 g; Fiber: 3 g; Protein: 34 g.

6.4 Cauliflower Fried Rice

Preparation time: 5 mins

Cooking time: 15 mins

Servings: 5

Ingredients:

- 2 tbsp. unsalted butter

- 1/2 large onion, finely diced

- 2 cloves garlic, minced

- 2 large eggs

- 1/2 medium red bell pepper, finely diced

- black pepper to taste

- sea salt to taste

- 2 tbsp. coconut aminos

- 1 medium head cauliflower

- 3 medium green onions, chopped

- 1 tsp. toasted sesame oil

Instructions:

- Take off the leaves and stems of the cauliflower. To make cauliflower rice, put the cauliflower florets into a food processor with grating attachment and process. You can also use a box grater to turn the cauliflower into rice.

- In a large sauté pan, melt a tablespoon of butter over medium heat. Add the red peppers, garlic, and onions. Saute the onions for about 8 to 10 minutes, until they are clear and just start turning brown.

- Mix the eggs with 1/2 tsp. of sea salt and a pinch of black pepper. Once the onions are done, move the vegetables to one side of the pan and a dd the eggs that have been whisked to the other side and cook them for a few minutes, until they are just about scrambled.

- Move everything back to the side of the pan and add the last tablespoon of butter. Once it melts, turn up the heat to medium-high, add the cauliflower right away, and stir everything to coat. Add black pepper and sea salt to taste. Stir fry the cauliflower for about 5 minutes, until they are soft but not mushy.

- Take the pan off the heat. Stir in the chopped green onions, coconut aminos, and sesame oil.

Nutritional values per serving: Calories 127 /kcal; Fat: 8 g; Carbs: 11 g; Fiber: 5 g; Protein: 5 g.

6.5 Keto Cabbage Rolls

Preparation time: 25 mins

Cooking time: 1 hour

Servings: 6

Ingredients:

- 1 head Cabbage

- 14.5-oz canned Diced tomatoes, drained

- 1 lb. Ground beef

- 4 cloves Garlic, minced

- 1 large Egg

- 1 tsp. Sea salt

- 2 tsp. Italian seasoning

- 1 cup Cauliflower rice

- 1/4 tsp. Black pepper

- 15-oz canned Tomato sauce

Instructions:

- Set the oven temperature to 350 degrees F.

- Bring water in a large pot to a boil. Put the whole head of cabbage into the water that is boiling. Boil for 5–8 minutes, or just until the leaves can be bend. They will turn a bright green color, and the leaves on the outside may fall off. This is fine, and you can remove them out.

- Take the cabbage out of the water and keep it aside to cool. Leave the boiled water in the pot for now. You might need it later when you are peeling the cabbage leaves.

- In the meantime, prepare the cauliflower rice mixture. Combine the ground beef, egg, diced tomatoes, Italian seasoning, minced garlic, black pepper, and sea salt in a large pan. Mix until everything is just mixed, but don't mix too much. Mix in the cauliflower and give it a mix. Set aside.

- Spread half of the tomato sauce in a large ceramic baking dish that is either rectangular or oval.

Set aside.

- Carefully remove the cabbage's leaves. To do this, turn the cabbage over so that the side with the core is facing up. Cut the leaves off the core one by one, and then carefully peel. Instead of peeling back the cabbage leaves, slide your fingers in between layers to pull them out. The outside of the leaves will be soft and easy to peel, but the inside may be more firm. If they are too hard and stiff to bend, you can put the half-peeled cabbage back into the boiling water for a few more minutes to soften them up more.

- Cut a "V" shape out of the thick rib in the middle of each cabbage leaf. On one end of a cabbage leaf, shape 1/3 cup of the beef mixture into a log. Like a burrito, fold the sides in and roll it up. Put the cabbage roll, seam side at base, on top of the sauce in the baking dish.

- Spread the cabbage rolls with the rest of the tomato sauce. Wrap foil tightly around the baking dish. Bake the rolls for 1 hour, or until they are fully cooked.

Nutritional values per serving: Calories 321 /kcal; Fat: 18 g; Carbs: 15 g; Fiber: 5 g; Protein: 25 g.

6.6 Creamed Spinach

Preparation time: 5 mins

Cooking time: 10 mins

Servings: 4

Ingredients:

- 3 tbsp. unsalted butter

- 10 oz. baby spinach

- 4 cloves garlic, minced

- 4 oz. cream cheese, cubed

- 1/2 cup heavy cream

- ¼ tsp. sea salt

- 1 tsp. Italian seasoning

- Parmesan cheese, for serving

- ¼ tsp. black pepper

Instructions:

- On medium heat, melt butter in a large pan with tall sides. Add minced garlic and cook it until it smells good.

- Add spinach. Saute for 2–4 minutes, until the leaves are wilted. If the pan is too packed to mix or you can't stuff all the spinach, add in a batch cover for 1–2 minutes. This will let the spinach at the bottom wilt. Then you can start to stir with a folding motion and add more in batches as needed.

- Add cream cheese, heavy cream, Italian seasoning, black pepper, and sea salt. Keep stirring until it thickens.

- Sprinkle Parmesan cheese on top and serve it as a side.

Nutritional values per serving: Calories 274 /kcal; Fat: 27 g; Carbs: 5 g; Fiber: 1 g; Protein: 4 g.

6.7 Cauliflower Tater Tots

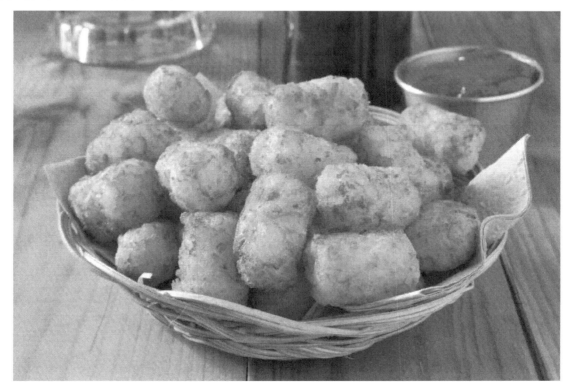

Preparation time: 10 mins

Cooking time: 20 mins

Servings: 3

Ingredients:

- 10 oz. cauliflower, riced

- ¾ cup mozzarella cheese, shredded

- ¼ tsp. white pepper powder

- ¼ cup coconut flour

- ¾ cup parmesan cheese, shredded

- ½ tsp. salt

- 1 large egg

Instructions:

- Turn the oven on to 425°F. Put parchment paper on a cookie sheet and set it aside.

- Put the cauliflower rice in a container that can go in the microwave, add the water, and cook for 3–5 minutes, until the cauliflower is fully cooked. Let it cool.

- When the cauliflower is cool enough to manage, put it in a clean kitchen towel or cloth and lightly squeeze it to get about half of the liquid out.

- Put the cauliflower and the rest of the ingredients into a bowl and mix well.

- Use a cookie scoop to quantify out the mixture, and then shape it with your hands. Set on your baking sheet.

- Spray olive oil cooking spray on the tater tots.

- After 10 minutes, change the tots' side and bake for a further 10-15 minutes.

- Serve hot and enjoy.

Nutritional values per serving: Calories 275 /kcal; Fat: 16 g; Carbs: 10 g; Fiber: 6 g; Protein: 21 g.

6.8 Mashed Cauliflower With Chives And Parmesan

Preparation time: 10 mins

Cooking time: 15 mins

Servings: 4

Ingredients:

- 2 small heads cauliflower, cut into florets

- 1/4 cup Parmesan cheese, grated

- Kosher salt to taste

- 2 cups chicken broth

- ¼ cup fresh chives, chopped

- ¼ tsp. black pepper

Instructions:

- Add the chicken broth and cauliflower and in a medium saucepan and bring to a boil. Turn the heat down to a simmer, cover, and cook for the cauliflower for 15–20 minutes, or until the cauliflower is soft but not falling apart.

- Transfer the cooked cauliflower to a blender or food processor and puree until smooth and silky.

- Transfer the cauliflower puree into a bowl and add the chopped chives and Parmesan in it. Season the mashed cauliflower with kosher salt and black pepper and serve.

Nutritional values per serving: Calories 33 /kcal; Fat: 2 g; Carbs: 1 g; Fiber: 0 g; Protein: 3 g.

6.9 Sushi Rolls Without Rice

Preparation time: 15 mins

Cooking time: 0 mins

Servings: 4

Ingredients:

- 4 oz. raw sushi grade fish or Smoked salmon

- ½ medium Cucumber

- ¼ large Red bell pepper

- 20 sheets Seaweed snacks

- ½ medium Avocado

Instructions:

- Cut the red peppers and cucumbers into thin slices like matchstick-sized, about 1/4 inches in width and as long as the narrow side of a seaweed snack sheet. Avocado and salmon should be cut into pieces that are the same length but wider. You'll need 20 of each kind.

- Set 5 seaweed snacks in a row on a cutting board in a single layer. Fill a nearby bowl with cold water. Wet Soak your finger by dipping it in water and wet the short corner of each sheet of seaweed. Put one piece of salmon, cucumber, red pepper, and avocado on the side of the first seaweed snack that is not facing you.

- Repeat step 2 until the whole row is done. When the entire row is done, wrap the first seaweed snack and push the edge to seal it. By the time you've finished adding the last piece, the wet edge of the first piece will have softened on its own. Place on a plate with the seam side down.

- Repeat steps 2 and 3 until all of the seaweed snack sheets are used up.

Nutritional values per serving: Calories 80 /kcal; Fat: 5 g; Carbs: 4 g; Fiber: 2 g; Protein: 6 g.

6.10 Shirataki Noodles

Preparation time: 5 mins

Cooking time: 20 mins

Servings: 4

Ingredients:

- 28 oz. shirataki noodles

- 4 cloves garlic, minced

- 1 tbsp. olive oil

- 2/3 cup heavy cream

- 2/3 cup chicken bone broth

- sea salt, to taste

- 1/2 cup grated parmesan cheese

- ¼ tsp. black pepper

Instructions:

- Shirataki noodles should be well rinsed in a colander with cool running water.

- Water should be heated up in a pot. Boil the konjac noodles for 3 minutes after adding them. Rinse well one more with running water.

- Dry the noodles well by patting.

- Over medium-high heat, preheat a sizable pan with a heavy bottom. Add the noodles and stir-fry for about 10 minutes, or until extremely dry, without adding any oil. To keep warm, take out the noodles and cover.

- Over medium heat, add olive oil to the skillet. When aromatic, add the minced garlic and simmer for about a minute.

- Add the cream and the broth. Turn up the heat to a simmer, then turn it down and simmer for about 5-7 minutes, or until the volume is cut in half.

- Add the parmesan cheese gradually and mix until smooth.

- Re-add the noodles to the skillet and toss with the sauce to coat. Cook until heated for 1-2 minutes. If necessary, season to taste with salt and pepper.

Nutritional values per serving: Calories 235 /kcal; Fat: 21 g; Carbs: 5 g; Fiber: 2 g; Protein: 8 g.

Chapter 7: Soups And Salads

7.1 Broccoli Cheese Soup

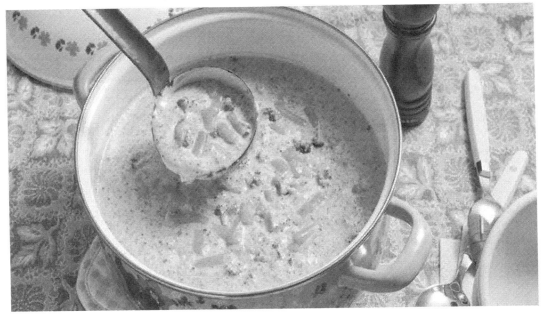

Preparation time: 5 mins

Cooking time: 15 mins

Servings: 5

Ingredients:

- 1 tbsp. butter

- ½ cup chopped onion

- 3 cloves garlic, minced

- 3 ½ cups chicken broth

- 3 cups broccoli florets

- 1/2 tsp. garlic powder

- 1 cup heavy cream

- salt and pepper, to taste

- ½ tsp. xanthan gum

- 3 cups shredded cheddar

Instructions:

- Cook the onion and garlic in the butter in a large pot over medium-high heat. Saute until fragrant. Into the pot, add the chicken broth, broccoli florets, and heavy cream. Season the soup with salt, garlic powder and pepper.

- Bring the soup to a boil, then turn the heat down to medium and let it cook for 10 minutes with the lid off.

- Take the pot off the heat and add 1 cup of shredded cheese at a time. Before adding the next cup of cheese, stir in each cup of cheese. This helps keep the soup from getting lumpy.

- Mix 1/2 tsp. of xanthan gum into the soup to make it thicker.

- Serve right away in small bowls with a little bit of shredded cheese on top.

Nutritional values per serving: Calories 514 /kcal; Fat: 43 g; Carbs: 12 g; Fiber: 3 g; Protein: 21 g.

7.2 Creamy Pumpkin Soup

Preparation time: 5 mins

Cooking time: 25 mins

Servings: 5

Ingredients:

- 2 tbsp. olive oil

- 2 cloves garlic, minced

- 1 small yellow onion, diced

- 13.5-oz full-fat coconut milk, canned

- 4 cups chicken broth, reduced sodium

- 1/2 tsp. nutmeg

- 15-oz can pumpkin puree

- 1/2 tsp. black pepper

- 1/2 tsp. sea salt

Instructions:

- On medium heat, heat the olive oil in a dutch oven. Add the onion and cook it for about 5 to 7 minutes, until it becomes clear.

- Add the garlic and cook it for a minute or two, until it smells good.

- Mix in the chicken broth, pumpkin, coconut milk, sea salt, nutmeg, and black pepper.

- Puree the soup with an immersion blender until it is creamy and smooth.

- Bring soup to a boil, then turn down the heat and let it simmer for about 25 to 30 minutes, until it's the right thickness and the flavors have developed.

Nutritional values per serving: Calories 242 /kcal; Fat: 22 g; Carbs: 11 g; Fiber: 3 g; Protein: 4 g.

7.3 Cauliflower Cheese Soup

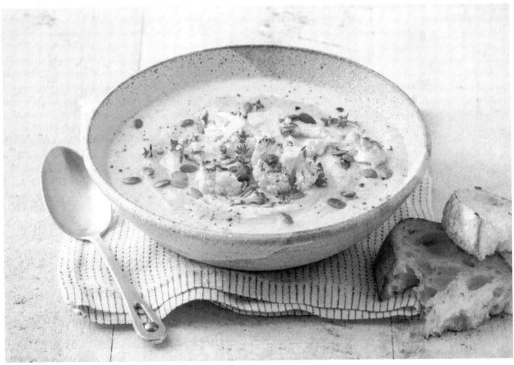

Preparation time: 5 mins

Cooking time: 20 mins

Servings: 8

Ingredients:

- 4 cups cauliflower florets

- 3 ½ cups chicken broth, reduced sodium

- 1 cup heavy cream

- 4 cloves garlic, minced

- 3 cups cheddar cheese, shredded

Instructions:

- Sauté the garlic in a dutch oven over medium heat for one minute, until it smells good.

- Mix in the cauliflower florets, heavy cream and chicken broth. Bring to a boil, then turn down the heat and let it simmer for 10–20 minutes, or until the cauliflower is soft.

- Take out about a third of the cauliflower pieces with a slotted spoon and set them aside.

- Blend the soup with the rest of the cauliflower with an immersion blender.

- Turn down the heat to low. Add cheese in batches 1/2 cup at a time while stirring, and keep stirring until the cheese melts. Blend it once more to make it smooth.

- Take the soup off the heat. Add the cauliflower florets that you saved back and serve warm.

Nutritional values per serving: Calories 298 /kcal; Fat: 25 g; Carbs: 6 g; Fiber: 1 g; Protein: 13 g.

7.4 Creamy Chicken Florentine Soup

Preparation time: 5 mins

Cooking time: 15 mins

Servings: 7

Ingredients:

- 1 tbsp. unsalted butter

- 1/2 large onion, diced

- 4 cloves garlic, minced

- 2 tsp. Italian seasoning

- 1 cup heavy cream

- 4 cups chicken broth, reduced sodium

- 10 oz. spinach

- 1 lb. shredded chicken

- sea salt to taste

- 14-oz can artichoke hearts

- ½ tsp. black pepper

Instructions:

- Melt the butter in a large pot over medium heat. Add in the garlic and fry it for about a minute, until fragrant.

- Add the onions and the Italian seasoning. Saute for 7 to 10 minutes, or until the food is slightly browned and just starting to get sweet. (You can sauté them longer if you want them to get more caramelized.)

- Add the cream, chicken broth, and spinach. For artichoke hearts, chop them up and add them. Add sea salt and black pepper at this point and bring to a , then simmer for about 5 minutes, till the spinach is soft and the soup is hot.

Nutritional values per serving: Calories 215 /kcal; Fat: 14 g; Carbs: 3 g; Fiber: 1 g; Protein: 16 g.

7.5 Homemade Vegetable Soup

Preparation time: 10 mins

Cooking time: 20 mins

Servings: 12

Ingredients:

- 2 tbsp. olive oil

- 2 large bell peppers, diced,

- 1 large onion, diced

- 1 medium head cauliflower, 1-inch florets

- 4 cloves garlic, minced

- 28 oz. diced tomatoes, canned

- 2 cups green beans, 1-inch pieces

- 1 tbsp. Italian seasoning

- 8 cups chicken broth, reduced sodium

- sea salt, to taste

- 2 dried bay leaves

- ¼ tsp. black pepper

Instructions:

- In a Dutch oven or pot, heat the olive oil over medium heat.

- Add the bell peppers and onions. Saute the onions and bell peppers for 7 to 10 minutes, until they are clear and browned.

- Add garlic and sauté for about 1 minute, until aromatic.

- Add the cauliflower, diced tomatoes, green beans, Italian seasoning, broth, and salt and pepper to taste.

- Add the bay leaves and get the soup boiling. Cover, turn the heat down to medium-low, and cook for about 10 to 20 minutes or until the vegetables are soft.

Nutritional values per serving: Calories 79 /kcal; Fat: 2 g; Carbs: 11 g; Fiber: 3 g; Protein: 2 g.

7.6 Cream Of Mushroom Soup

Preparation time: 10 mins

Cooking time: 30 mins

Servings: 5

Ingredients:

- 1 tbsp. olive oil

- 20 oz. mushrooms, sliced

- 1/2 medium onion, diced

- 2 cup chicken broth, reduced sodium

- 6 cloves garlic, minced

- 1 cup unsweetened almond milk

- 1 cup heavy cream

- ¼ tsp. black pepper

- ¾ tsp. sea salt

Instructions:

- In a large pot or Dutch oven, heat the olive oil over medium heat. Add the mushrooms and onions and cook them in the oil for 10 to 15 minutes, stirring every so often, until they are soft and lightly browned.

- Add the garlic and cook it for about a minute or until it starts to smell good.

- Mix in the chicken broth, almond milk, cream, black pepper and sea salt. Bring to a boil, then let it simmer for about 15 minutes, stirring every so often, until the flavors are just the way you like them.

- Use a stick blender to make a smooth puree.

Nutritional values per serving: Calories 233 /kcal; Fat: 21 g; Carbs: 7 g; Fiber: 2 g; Protein: 7 g.

7.7 Kale Crunch Salad

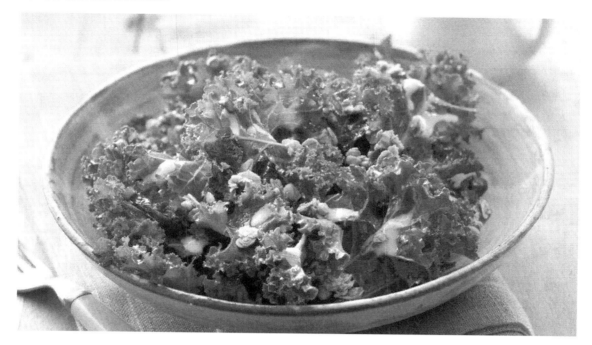

Preparation time: 10 mins

Cooking time: 0 mins

Servings: 6

Ingredients:

- 1/2 cup dried cranberries, sugar-free

- 3 tbsp. Eaton hemp hearts

- 5 oz. curly kale, chopped

- 3 tbsp. keto maple syrup

- 3 tbsp. almonds, sliced

- 1 tbsp. Dijon mustard

- 1½ tbsp. apple cider vinegar

- 1/8 tsp. black pepper

- 1/4 tsp. sea salt

- 1/4 cup olive oil

Instructions:

- Whisk the vinegar, maple syrup, salt, mustard, and pepper together in a small bowl. Pour the olive oil in it in a thin stream while whisking constantly until the ingredients are mixed together.

- Chop the kale and put it in a large bowl. Pour the dressing over the kale and rub it with your hands for 2 to 3 minutes, until the kale is soft.

- Add the almonds, cranberries, and hemp hearts. Toss and serve.

Nutritional values per serving: Calories 152 /kcal; Fat: 14 g; Carbs: 5 g; Fiber: 2 g; Protein: 4 g.

7.8 Creamy Cucumber Salad With Sour Cream

Preparation time: 10 minutes

Cooking time: 0 mins

Servings: 6

Ingredients:

- ½ cup sour cream

- 1 tbsp. olive oil

- ½ tsp. garlic powder

- ¼ tsp. black pepper

- 1 small red onion, sliced

- 2 tbsp. fresh dill, chopped

- 1 tbsp. lemon juice

- ½ tsp. sea salt

- 24 oz. cucumbers, sliced

Instructions:

- Whisk the sour cream, olive oil, dill, and garlic powder and lemon juice together in a large bowl. Add black pepper and sea salt to taste.

- Mix in the chopped red onions and cucumbers.

Nutritional values per serving: Calories 86 /kcal; Fat: 6 g; Carbs: 7 g; Fiber: 1 g; Protein: 2 g.

7.9 Healthy Avocado Tuna Salad

Preparation time: 10 mins

Cooking time: 0 mins

Servings: 4

Ingredients:

- 2 medium avocados

- 20 oz. canned tuna

- 2 tbsp. lime juice

- 3 tbsp. celery, finely chopped

- ¼ cup fresh cilantro, chopped

- 1 tbsp. jalapeños

- 3 tbsp. red onion, minced

- ½ tsp. sea salt, to taste

Instructions:

- Mash the lime juice, avocado, and sea salt together.

- Mix in the tuna, red onion, cilantro, jalapeño and celery. Mix everything together, breaking up any big pieces of tuna as needed.

- Adjust salt according to taste if needed. Serve right away.

Nutritional values per serving: Calories 169 /kcal; Fat: 14 g; Carbs: 10 g; Fiber: 6 g; Protein: 27 g.

7.10 Egg Salad

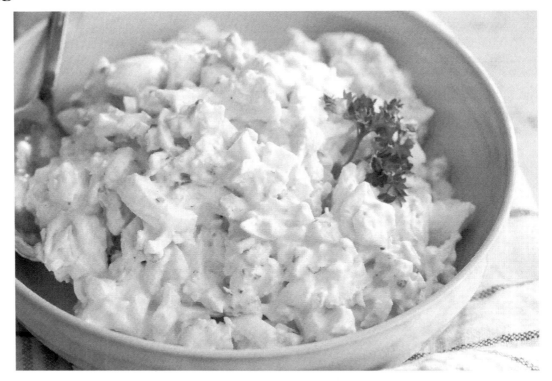

Preparation time: 5 mins

Cooking time: 0 mins

Servings: 4

Ingredients:

- 1/2 cup mayonnaise

- ¼ cup celery, finely chopped

- 8 large hard boiled eggs, diced

- 2 tbsp. chives, chopped

- 2 tbsp. white onion, minced

- 1/8 tsp. black pepper

- 1 tbsp. lemon juice

- 1 tbsp. Dijon mustard

- 1/2 tsp. sea salt

- paprika, for garnish

Instructions:

- Whisk the mayonnaise, lemon juice and mustard together in a medium bowl until smooth.

- Mix the eggs, onions, and chives in the prepared dressing. Add salt and pepper and sprinkle paprika on top.

Nutritional values per serving: Calories 362 /kcal; Fat: 32 g; Carbs: 2 g; Fiber: 0.4 g; Protein: 13 g.

Chapter 8: Dessert Recipes

8.1 Basic Orange Cheesecake

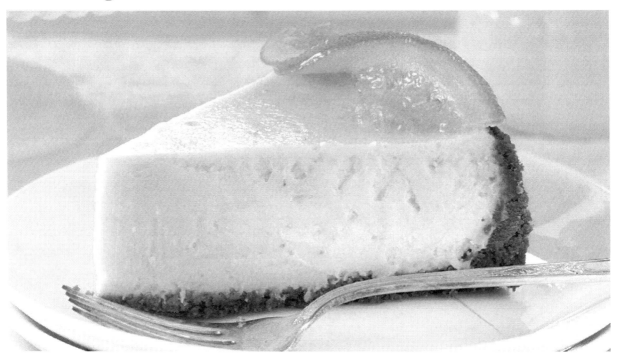

Preparation time: 15 minutes

Cooking time: 0 minutes

Servings: 12

Ingredients:

- 3 tbsp. Swerve

- 1 stick butter, room temperature

- 1 cup almond flour

- 1/2 cup unsweetened coconut, shredded Filling

- 1 tsp. powdered gelatin

- 17 oz. mascarpone cream

- 2 tbsp. orange juice

Instructions:

- Combine 1 tbsp. severe, 1 stick butter, 1 cup almond flour, and 1/2 cup unsweetened coconut for the crust thoroughly, and then press the dough into a baking dish that has been lightly oiled. Place it in the refrigerator to cool.

- Then, stir gelatin into 1 cup of hot water until all of it has dissolved. Add 1 cup of ice-cold water.

- Blend in the mascarpone cheese, orange juice, and 2 tbsp. Swerve until consistent and smooth. On top of the prepared crust, pour the filling. Enjoy!

Nutritional values per serving: Calories: 150 /kcal; Fat: 15 g; Carbs: 2 g; Fiber: 1 g; Protein: 2 g.

8.2 Cherry Ripe Slice

Preparation time: 30 mins + chilling time

Cooking time: 0 mins

Servings: 15

Ingredients:

Base

- 3.5 oz. shredded coconut, unsweetened

- 3.5 oz. almond flour

- 2 oz. Unsalted Butter

- 1 tbsp. Swerve

- 3.5 oz. Sugar Free Chocolate Chips

Filling

- 8 oz. Cream Cheese softened

- 1 tsp. cherry essence

- 2 oz. Swerve

- 3 tsp. gelatin

- 11 oz. Heavy Cream

- 3-4 drops red food coloring red

- 1/4 cup boiling water

Topping

- 3.5 oz. Sugar Free Chocolate Chips

- 1 tbsp. Heavy Cream

- 4 drops cherry essence

- 2 tsp. shredded coconut, unsweetened

- 4 drops Stevia, optional

Instructions:

Base

- Mix the shredded coconut, almond flour and Swerve in a bowl.

- Put the chocolate and butter in a separate bowl, and put that bowl over a pan of water that is slowly boiling. Make sure that the boiling water does not touch the bowl.

- Melt the chocolate and butter, and then mix them well with the dry ingredients.

- Press the base firmly and evenly into a 9x13 brownie pan.

- Put in the refrigerator to firm up while you make the next layer.

Filling

- With the whisk attachment on your stand mixer, whisk the cream cheese, swerve and cherry extract. Mix until it's smooth.

- Mix well after adding 2/3 of the heavy cream.

- In a separate bowl take the 1/4 cup of boiling water and add gelatin in it.

- Slowly add the gelatin mixture into your stand mixer while the mixer is going at a low speed.

- Add the rest of the cream and mix well until everything is smooth and well blended.

- Spoon two-third of the mixture over the chilled base.

- Mix well after adding the food coloring to the rest of the mixture.

- Put the pink mixture on top of the base and swirl it.

- Put it in the fridge for 3 hours, or better yet, leave it there overnight.

- Cut the dessert into squares and put them on a wooden board or a large dish.

Topping

- Mix the cherry essence and chocolate in a bowl.

- Place the bowl over a pot of water that is simmering, but don't let the bowl touch the water.

- When the chocolate melts, mix in the cream and stevia.

- Warm the chocolate and put it in a piping bag with a very fine tip. Drizzle the chocolate over the bars that have been put in the fridge.

- You can eat them right away, or you can cover them and put them in the fridge for up to a week.

Nutritional values per serving: Calories 306 /kcal; Fat: 28 g; Carbs: 5 g; Fiber: 3 g; Protein: 5 g.

8.3 Classic Cheesecake

Preparation time: 10 mins

Cooking time: 1 hour

Servings: 16

Ingredients:

- 2 cups almond flour

- 1 ¼ cups + 2 tbsp. powdered fruit allulose blend, divided

- 1/3 cup unsalted butter

- 32 oz. cream cheese, softened

- 2 tsp. vanilla extract, divided

- 1 tbsp. lemon juice

- 3 large eggs

Instructions:

- Set the oven temperature to 350°F. Line a spring form pan that is 9 inches across with parchment paper.

- To make the almond flour cheesecake crust, mix the chickpea flour, 2 tbsp. fruit allulose blend, melted butter, and 1 tsp. vanilla extract in a medium bowl until everything is well mixed. The dough will have some crumbles.

- Press the dough down into the bottom of the pan that has been set up. Bake for about 10–12 minutes, or until the top just turns golden. Leave it aside to cool at least 10 minutes.

- In the meantime, beat the 1 1/4 cups fruit allulose blend and cream cheese together on low to medium speed until fluffy. Now start beating eggs in this mixture on at a time.

- Mix in the vanilla extract and lemon juice. (Keep the mixer on low to medium speed the whole time. Too high a speed will add several air bubbles, which we don't want.)

- Put the filling on top of the crust in the pan. Use a spatula to smooth the top. Tap the pan on the kitchen shelf a few times to make sure there are no air bubbles.

- Bake for about 40–55 minutes, or until the center is almost set but still jiggly.

- Take the cake out of the oven. If the edges are locked to the pan, run a knife all around edge. Let the pan cool to room temperature on the counter, and then put it in the fridge for at least 4 hours, or better yet, overnight, until it is completely set.

Nutritional values per serving: Calories 325 /kcal; Fat: 31 g; Carbs: 6 g; Fiber: 1 g; Protein: 7 g.

8.4 Chocolate Fat Bombs

Preparation time: 10 mins

Cooking time: 0 mins

Servings: 20

Ingredients:

- 2 cup Macadamia nuts, dry roasted, salted

- 2 tbsp. MCT oil

- 2 tbsp. Coconut oil, melted

- 1/3 cup Powdered Monk Fruit Allulose Blend

- 1 tsp. Vanilla extract

- 3 tbsp. Macadamia nuts, crushed

- ¼ cup Cocoa powder

Instructions:

- Pulse macadamia nuts in a food processor or high-powered blender until they are mostly broken up into small pieces.

- Add MCT oil, vanilla essence and melted coconut oil. Puree the nuts until you get nut butter. (Try to make it smooth, but don't worry if there are some stray pieces.) If you need to, scrape down the sides.

- Add the sweetener and cocoa powder slowly, a couple of tablespoons at a time. Mix after each addition, until the mixture is smooth.

- Use parchment paper to line a mini muffin tin. Spoon or pour the batter into each liner until it's full, making sure it's even.

- On top of fat bombs, use the crushed macadamia nuts for garnish.

- Freeze the chocolate fat bombs for at least 30 minutes, until solid.

Nutritional values per serving: Calories 122 /kcal; Fat: 13 g; Carbs: 2 g; Fiber: 1 g; Protein: 1 g.

8.5 Red Velvet Cake

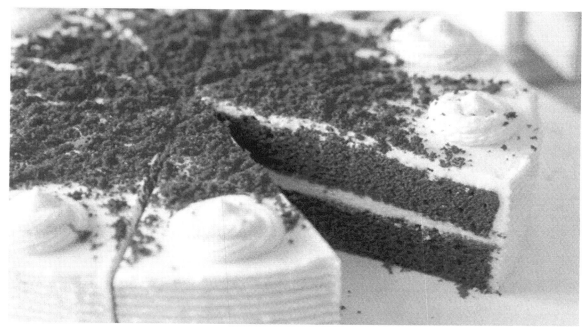

Preparation time: 10 mins

Cooking time: 35 mins

Servings: 24

Ingredients:

- 1½ cups fruit allulose blend

- 3 eggs, room temperature

- ¾ cup salted butter, softened

- ¾ cup sour cream, room temperature

- 1 tbsp. vanilla extract

- 1 tsp. white vinegar

- ½ cup unsweetened almond milk, room temperature

- 2 tbsp. cocoa powder

- 3 cups almond flour

- 2 tbsp. beet root powder

- 2 tsp. baking soda

- 3 ½ cups keto cream cheese frosting

- chopped pecans, for topping

Instructions:

- Set the oven temperature to 350 degrees F. Put parchment paper on the bottom of two 9-inch spring form pans.

- Beat fruit allulose blend and butter together in a large bowl until fluffy.

- One egg at a time beat in the eggs. Stir in the sour cream, vanilla, almond milk, and vinegar to avoid splashing. Then, beat the mixture to mix it all together.

- Slow down the mixer and add the almond flour 1/2 cup at a time, beating after each addition. Mix in the baking soda and cocoa powder until the batter is smooth. If you want to use beet root powder, beat it in one teaspoon at a time until you get the color you want.

- Split the dough between the two pans, and use a spatula to smooth the top. Bake for about 25 minutes, or until a toothpick that is stuck in the middle comes out clean. Let them cool all the way in the pans, then run a knife along the edges and flip them over to get them out.

- Put one layer of cake on a plate or cake stand. Use 3/4 cup frosting to cover the top. Place the second layer on top and add another 3/4 cup of frosting to the top. Then, use 1 1/2 cups frosting to frost the sides. Add chopped pecans on top and serve.

Nutritional values per serving: Calories 286 /kcal; Fat: 27 g; Carbs: 5 g; Fiber: 2 g; Protein: 5 g.

8.6 Apple Pie

Preparation time: 25 mins

Cooking time: 1 hour 10 mins

Servings: 12

Ingredients:

Filling

- 1/4 cup powdered fruit allulose blend

- 1/2 cup unsalted butter

- 2 tsp. cinnamon

- 6 tbsp. lemon juice, divided

- 1/2 tsp. cardamom

- 1 tsp. nutmeg

- 1 tbsp. unflavored gelatin powder

- 1 tsp. vanilla extract

- 5 medium apples, diced

- 1/2 tsp. maple extract

Crust

- 1/3 cup Besti monk fruit allulose blend

- 3¾ cups almond flour

- 1/2 cup unsalted butter, melted

- 1/2 tsp. sea salt

- 1/2 tsp. vanilla extract

- 1 large egg

- 2 tbsp. water

- 1 tbsp. unflavored gelatin powder

Instructions:

Filling

- Mix 3 tablespoons of lemon juice with the gelatin powder in a small bowl. Leave it aside to bloom.

- Melt the butter in a large, 3.5-quart pot over medium heat. Stir in the remaining 3 tbsp. of lemon juice, the powdered sweetener, the nutmeg, cinnamon, and cardamom. When the gelatin mixture has bloomed, whisk it into the pan until it has dissolved.

- Put the apple cubes in the pan. Bring to a low boil. Simmer over medium heat for 30 to 40 minutes, until the apple is very soft and the mixture is thick like apple pie filling.

- Add the maple and vanilla extracts and mix them in.

- Set the filling aside for at least 20 minutes to cool until it is no hotter than lukewarm.

Crust

- In the meantime, heat the oven to 350°F.

- Mix the almond flour, sea salt and Besti together in a large bowl.

- Stir in the egg and melted butter until everything is well mixed. Before adding it to the dry ingredients, stir the vanilla into the melted butter. The "dough" will be dry and break apart easily. Just keep stirring, pressing, and mixing it until it's all the same and there's no more almond flour powder.

- Mix water and gelatin powder, and mix them together with a hand mixer until everything is the same.

- Cut the dough in two. Press half of the dough into the bottom and up the sides of the pie pan that has been greased. Set aside the second half of the dough.

- Bake the crust for 10 to 12 minutes, or until it is just barely golden.

- Set it aside for at least 10 minutes to cool down before adding the filling.

- Put the other half of the dough between two pieces of parchment paper that have been lightly oiled. For the top crust, use a rolling pin and parchment paper to make a circle that is just a little bit bigger than the top of the pie pan.

Assembling

- If the oven has cooled, heat it back up to 350°F. Before putting the pie together, make sure the bottom crust and filling are neither too hot nor too cold.

- Move the filling carefully to the bottom crust that has already cooled.

- Take off the top piece of parchment paper from the top crust that has been rolled out. Using the bottom piece of parchment paper, quickly and carefully flip the top crust over onto the pie. Then, gently peel off the parchment paper. Cut off any extra top crust around the edges with a knife. Make sure the top crust still covers the bottom crust completely. Press the edges down with your fingers to seal them. Cut four slits in the pie top.

- Bake for 20 to 25 minutes, or until the edges are browned. Cover the pie's edges with foil and bake for another 5 to 15 minutes, until the upper crust is light golden and almost firm. (It won't be fully firm until it cools down.)

- Take the pie out of the oven and let it cool completely before you try to cut it or take it out of the pan.

Nutritional values per serving: Calories 363 /kcal; Fat: 33 g; Carbs: 12 g; Fiber: 4 g; Protein: 10 g.

8.7 Crustless Pumpkin Pie

Preparation time: 10 mins

Cooking time: 35 mins

Servings: 8

Ingredients:

- 15-oz. can pumpkin puree

- 3 large eggs, room temperature

- ½ cup heavy cream

- ¼ cup brown fruit allulose blend

- 1 tbsp. pumpkin pie spice

- ½ cup powdered fruit allulose blend

- 1/2 tbsp. vanilla extract

- 1/4 tsp. sea salt

- 2 tsp. unflavored gelatin powder

Instructions:

- Set the oven temperature to 300°F. Use butte cooking spray to grease a pie pan.

- Mix the cream, pumpkin, eggs, Besti Brown, pumpkin pie spice, Besti Powdered, sea salt and vanilla with a hand mixer on medium-low speed in a large bowl until smooth.

- Sprinkle the gelatin powder on the batter, and then beat it right away until it is all the same color. Give the batter a 5 minute break.

- Fill a pie pan with the batter. Tap on the counter gently to get rid of any air bubbles.

- Bake the pumpkin pie without a crust for 35 to 45 minutes, or until the center is almost set but still moves a little when you shake the pan. With a meat thermometer, the internal temperature should be between 165 and 170°F.

- Let it cool completely on the kitchen shelf, uncovered, before putting it in the fridge for at least 2 hours or overnight.

Nutritional values per serving: Calories 104 /kcal; Fat: 7 g; Carbs: 5 g; Fiber: 2 g; Protein: 4 g.

8.8 Pumpkin Roll

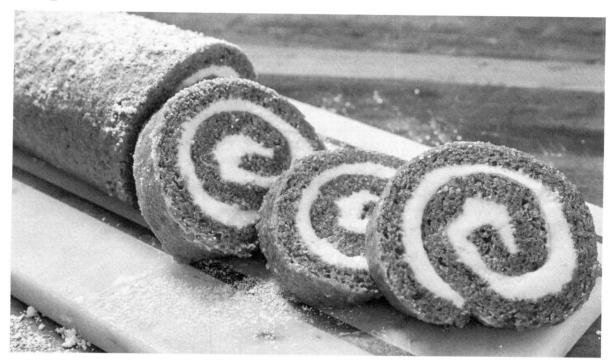

Preparation time: 10 mins + chilling time

Cooking time: 30 mins

Servings: 10

Ingredients:

Cake

- 4 tbsp. Wholesome Yum Coconut Flour

- 1 cup Almond Flour

- 1/4 tsp. Sea salt

- 1 tsp. Baking powder

- 1/2 cup Besti Monk Fruit Allulose Blend

- 1 tsp. Xanthan gum

- 4 large Eggs

- 1 tsp. Pumpkin pie spice

- 1 tsp. Vanilla extract

- 2/3 cup Pumpkin puree

Filling

- 8 oz. Cream cheese, softened

- 2 tbsp. Unsalted butter, softened

- 1 tsp. Vanilla extract

- 1/4 cup Powdered Fruit Allulose Blend

Instructions:

Cake

- Set oven temperature to 350°F.

- Mix the coconut flour, almond flour, xanthan gum, baking powder, Besti, sea salt, and pumpkin pie spice together in a large bowl.

- Whisk the eggs, vanilla and pumpkin puree in a small bowl.

- Mix the dry ingredients into the wet ones until they are completely mixed in.

- Wrap parchment paper around a 913-inch pan and spray the paper with cooking spray. Spread the cake batter out in an even layer on the whole cookie sheet.

- Bake for 10 to 13 minutes, or until the cake bounces back when touched and a toothpick inserted into the middle comes out clean. Set aside and wait 10 minutes for it to cool down a bit.

- Roll the cake tightly using the short side of the parchment paper, and let it cool for another 30 minutes.

Cream cheese filling

- In the meantime, make cream cheese filling by mixing Cream cheese, unsalted butter, vanilla extract and powdered Fruit Allulose Blend in a large bowl using electric mixer for 5 minutes until everything is well combined.

Assembling

- Once the cake is completely cool, carefully unroll it so it doesn't break. Spread the filling on the cake, leaving a 1-inch space around the edges.

- Roll the cake back up with the parchment paper, keeping it intact but not so tight that it breaks and the filling spills out. Before cutting, put in the fridge for at least an hour, but preferably overnight.

Nutritional values per serving: Calories 214 /kcal; Fat: 18 g; Carbs: 7 g; Fiber: 3 g; Protein: 7 g.

8.9 Coconut Flour Cake

Preparation time: 20 mins

Cooking time: 20 mins

Servings: 12

Ingredients:

Cake

- 1 cup unsalted butter, softened

- 6 large eggs, room temperature

- ¾ cup coconut milk beverage

- 2 cups Besti monk fruit allulose blend

- ½ tbsp. vanilla extract

- ¾ cup sour cream

- 1 tbsp. baking powder

- 1½ cups wholesome yum coconut flour

- ¼ tsp. sea salt

Frosting

- 1½ cups unsalted butter, softened

- 1 tsp. vanilla extract

- 1 cup Besti powdered fruit allulose blend

- 1 tbsp. heavy cream

- 1/8 tsp. sea salt

Topping

- 1 cup Unsweetened coconut flakes

Instructions:

Cake

- Set the oven temperature to 350°F. Put parchment paper at the base of two 9-inch spring form pans.

- In a large bowl, beat the butter and Besti sweetener with a hand mixer on medium speed for 3 minutes, until the mixture is light in color and fluffy.

- One egg at a time beat in the eggs. Mix in the sour cream, coconut milk, and vanilla extract.

- Mix in the baking powder, salt, and coconut flour until the batter is smooth.

- Use a spatula to smooth the tops of the two cake pans with the dough. Bake for about 20 minutes, moving the pan halfway through if necessary, or until a toothpick inserted into the center comes out clean. Let the layers of coconut flour cake cool all the way in the pans before taking them out.

Frosting

- Mix the Butter and Besti together with a hand mixer for 2 to 3 minutes, until the mixture is fluffy and light yellow. (Start at a low speed and then speed up after adding the sweetener.)

- Slowly beat in the vanilla, cream, and salt.

- Turn the mixer up to high and beat for two to three minutes, or until the consistency you want is reached.

Assembling

- On a cake stand, put one layer of cake. Use 3/4 cup frosting to cover the top. Put the second cake layer on top and frost it with 3/4 cup more frosting. Last, use the rest of the frosting to frost the sides.

- Put the coconut flakes in a large pan over medium heat and toast them until golden, about 2 minutes. Decorate the top and sides of the cake using toasted coconut that has already been frosted.

Nutritional values per serving: Calories 316 /kcal; Fat: 27 g; Carbs: 12 g; Fiber: 6 g; Protein: 6 g.

8.10 Almond Butter Cookies

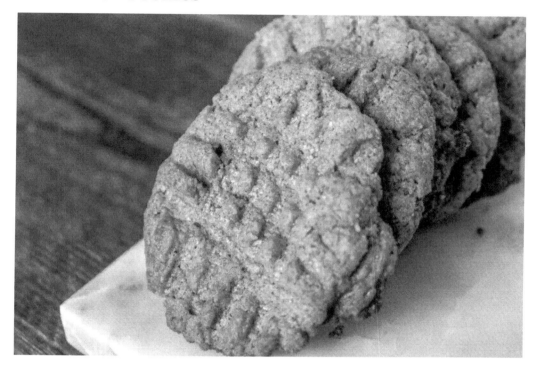

Preparation time: 5 mins

Cooking time: 15 mins

Servings: 12

Ingredients:

- 1¼ cups almond butter

- 1/3 cup Besti monk fruit allulose blend

- 1 tsp vanilla extract, optional

- 2 large eggs

- ¼ tsp. sea salt, optional

Instructions:

- Set the oven temperature to 350°F. Put parchment paper on a cookie sheet.

- Mix all the ingredients together in a large bowl until they are well mixed.

- Using a medium cookie scoop, put 12 balls of dough on the cookie sheet that has been prepared. Use a fork to make a crisscross pattern on the dough. To keep the fork from getting stuck, dip it in a cup of cold water between each cookie and wipe it clean with a paper towel.

- Bake for 15-20 minutes, until light golden from top. Let the cookies cool down all the way before taking them off the baking sheet. As the cookies cool, they will get firmer.

Nutritional values per serving: Calories 176 /kcal; Fat: 15 g; Carbs: 5 g; Fiber: 3 g; Protein: 7 g.

21 Days Meal plan

Day 1

Breakfast: Ham, mushroom and spinach frittata

Lunch: Crockpot Curry Chicken

Dinner: Shrimp Scampi with Zucchini Noodles

Day 2

Breakfast: Tomato Baked Eggs

Lunch: Chicken Parmesan

Dinner: Beef Stew

Day 3

Breakfast: Mushroom Brunch

Lunch: Thai Beef Curry

Dinner: Chipotle Beef Barbacoa

Day 4

Breakfast: Omelette Roll-Up

Lunch: Spinach Stuffed Chicken Breast

Dinner: Lamb Korma

Day 5

Breakfast: Vegetable Frittata

Lunch: Chicken Fajita Casserole

Dinner: Moroccan Meatballs

Day 6

Breakfast: Cauliflower Fritters

Lunch: Beef Stroganoff

Dinner: Creamy Tuscan Chicken

Day 7

Breakfast: Savory Zucchini Muffins

Lunch: Orange Chicken

Dinner: Beef Stew

Day 8

Breakfast: Carnivore Eggs

Lunch: Philly Cheesesteak Casserole

Dinner: Creamy Dijon Chicken

Day 9

Breakfast: Breakfast Casserole

Lunch: Crustless Ham and Swiss Quiche

Dinner: Lemon Butter Baked Tilapia

Day 10

Breakfast: Breakfast Sandwich

Lunch: Creamy Lemon Chicken

Dinner: Steak and Shrimp

Day 11

Breakfast: Ham, mushroom and spinach frittata

Lunch: Blue Cheese Pork Medallions

Dinner: Blackened Tilapia with Zucchini Noodles

Day 12

Breakfast: Omelette Roll-Up

Lunch: Orange Chicken

Dinner: Chipotle Beef Barbacoa

Day 13

Breakfast: Breakfast Casserole

Lunch: Beef Stroganoff

Dinner: Lamb Korma

Day 14

Breakfast: Savory Zucchini Muffins

Lunch: Chicken Bacon Ranch Casserole

Dinner: Eggplant Lasagna

Day 15

Breakfast: Vegetable Frittata

Lunch: Thai Beef Curry

Dinner: Cheeseburger Casserole

Day 16

Breakfast: Carnivore Eggs

Lunch: Chicken Fajita Casserole

Dinner: Lemon Butter Baked Tilapia

Day 17

Breakfast: Savory Zucchini Muffins

Lunch: Crockpot Curry Chicken

Dinner: Moroccan Meatballs

Day 18

Breakfast: Omelette Roll-Up

Lunch: Chicken Parmesan

Dinner: Eggplant Lasagna

Day 19

Breakfast: Breakfast Sandwich

Lunch: Chicken Bacon Ranch Casserole

Dinner: Steak and Shrimp

Day 20

Breakfast: Mushroom Brunch

Lunch: Spinach Stuffed Chicken Breast

Dinner: Shrimp Scampi with Zucchini Noodles

Day 21

Breakfast: Tomato Baked Eggs

Lunch: Blue Cheese Pork Medallions

Dinner: Creamy Tuscan Chicken

Conclusion

One of the most important parts of any diet or change in lifestyle has always been the recipes that fit with the diet's principles. There are many ways to get your body into ketosis and lose weight. But you definitely don't want to get there by eating the same old dishes all the time.

Variety is the talk of the town here, which is important for making sure the ketogenic diet, will last. This step-by-step keto cookbook has lots of tasty and flavorful recipes that will help anyone on a keto diet, no matter where they are in their journey.

If you are just starting out with keto and you got this recipe book, it will help you a lot as you go along. There are multiple recipes, so you can pick and choose the ones that sound best to you.